# THE FOURTH STATE OF CONSCIOUSNESS

How to Reach Turiya

Author: Ishan Kyan

Copyright @ 2021 by Ishan Kyan

# Table of Contents

Chapter One  Introduction ................................................................ 1

Chapter Two  What Are the Four States of Consciousness? ........... 3

Chapter Three  Understanding Turiya ........................................... 10

Chapter Four  The Upanishad ........................................................ 34

Chapter Five  The Conscious Mind ............................................... 49

Chapter Six  Meditation ................................................................ 55

Chapter Seven  Understanding the Mind. .................................... 64

Chapter Eight  Phenomenology, Experiences, and States of Consciousness ............................................................................... 73

Chapter Nine  Understanding the Body of Man ........................... 85

Chapter Ten  Conclusions ............................................................ 102

# Chapter One

# Introduction

Yoga secret is part of our everyday lives, concealed within our own natural patterns & behaviour– how, in the days, months, seasons and years, we see, perceive, talk and breathe. Perhaps the greatest mysteries are our current state of consciousness and its various levels.

Consciousness is the very foundation of our life, and remains as the persistent inner light behind outward life changes. By nature, we are conscious beings who work with the resources of mind and body. In our accumulation of knowledge across the realms of time and space, our present Embodiment is just another one. Awareness gives us our thinking, thinking and knowledge, which are the inner truth from which body and mind operate. It is the heart of our life.

Nevertheless, we are largely unaware of the meaning of our consciousness. We are so busy with our understanding of the outside world that we have completely forgotten its roots. Our challenging lives preclude us from understanding who we are, what (if anything) death survives and what our ultimate aim is. We are caught in our own physical image, losing our inner meaning of colors. Our transient lives conceal our inner link to the Eternal.

The effect of these distracting is that we are guided by outside influences rather than internal awareness through confusion, desire and sorrow. We stay at our tumultuous surface and seldom come to the quiet depths of our being. In the thick, material world, we seek outer fulfilment and neglect the hidden happiness that resides in us.

The mystery of consciousness and its development is our lives. This is our key thing to learn. We ought to be driven to research our own minds carefully, not just the outside world. We will explore the profound consequences of the regular movements of our consciousness by waking and sleeping in the search of self-knowledge. In the Indian spiritual tradition such review was long established, as the pages before us indicate.

Dreams are often considered to be delusional, unreal and meaningless to everyday life. Yes, there's much more that we are told to dream and sleep in the west. Indian spiritual awareness gives an insight of dreams that can help us live a rich, more conscious life.

# Chapter Two

# What Are the Four States of Consciousness?

Consciousness is not simply a question of metaphysics that is little practical for us. This is the origin and the foundation of all our lives. The Sages in India realized that every day is a journey through consciousness, because they spoke of four states: waking, dreaming, deep sleep and a fourth state beyond (technically called "Non-REM sleep."). They are usually interested only in the waking state, but also in the sense, identification, and perceptions of dreams and deep sleep. The two subtle states, from wellbeing to spirituality, have a profound impact on us and should not be ignored.

The Waking State, Jagrat Avantha

Throughout the day we do not live in a single state of mind. By waking, dreaming and deep sleep the essence of our consciousness radically changes. The waking state shows us through the five senses a vivid outside world. Each of us can sense it consistently and strongly. It seems objective. However, we have several variations from moments of clarity to periods of confusion and dullness in relation to our feelings, emotions and attention spans. Therefore, physical experiences by themselves have many changes, uneasiness and are ultimately temporary.

## Dreaming, Svapna Avastha

The dream state provides a vivid, vibrant, rapidly changing, and subjective, inner consciousness. We construct our own personal reality in our visions, with a sense of time and space but with a seemingly unsustainable impact on our exterior lives. Typically, as contrasted with the truth we offer to the waking world, we regard this dream world as unreal. Nevertheless, visions and astral encounters are beautiful and fascinating.

Many of us find the dream state simply a framework for repercussion and communicating our memories and subconscious patterns. Such practices are mostly pointless, but we have meaningful dreams at times. We have dreams that enrich our waking life, always inspiring. Or maybe we have disturbing dreams that lead us to fear the state of dreaming. A dream state review shows just representation of the stresses and traumas in the waking state. Psychoanalytical science His work is confined to the unconscious and unconscious states of consciousness, with little knowledge of more complex levels of consciousness beyond that.

Dreaming is not only Dreaming; it's true, it's important. For explanations, you can't dream. There's a causality even of a dream. It's significant, it tells you something. Instead, it tells more about you and reveals more when you're big, because if you're waking you and others can deceive yourself and others, but you can't disappoint your dreams. Dreams are harder because we have not yet found a system for dreaming and dreaming with masks. The dreams are still naked, genuine; they show more truly the real face when you are awake than anyone you use.

We are often fantasized overall, suggesting that we dream even in waking conditions. This moves too slowly for us to see our waking state, and does not give us the sort of desire that we are looking for. This makes it a fascinating hobby to explore the realms of creativity and vision. The technology today gives us "virtual reality" and "increased world" that are very much like waking dream projections. Man will soon prefer this virtual reality, somewhere between waking and sleeping, as it can help fulfil our dreams and desires but it is stronger than the dream state than physical reality. Some scientific miracles are now supernatural approaching.

Yoga tells us that there is a whole universe of dreams and we have our own life and personality. It is our astral body that remains in our soul after our experience of death. While we also live in the astral body continuously, many people are only superficially conscious of it, but some souls have a deep astral presence all their days. Many such self-conscious people are musicians, mystics, occultists and psychics.

We function with a goal-orientated universe of collective karma during the waking cycle. In the state of dreaming, we function with a fictional world that comes from our thoughts and imaginations. That presents us with a dilemma. If we are unable to control our minds, dreaming can easily become bad dreams, nights or ties to low-astral worlds of chaos, violence, desire, anger and hate. Our dream world will remain chaotic without control of our emotions.

Deep Sleep, Sushupti Avastha

Deep sleep draws us into a realm of unmanifest awareness that obscures everything and takes it back to its grazing form. Deep sleep is easy to overlook, but it serves as the basis and support for waking and dreaming conditions in which it can not function.

We are looking forward to our last state of rest and recovery as we sleep.

During deeper sleep we all sense peace, relaxation and regeneration in the heart. In this state, we are not conscious of ourselves but only preserve its meaning or rasa. We are waking up with the feeling of night. Deep sleep is a peaceful sleep, where we experience joy naturally in our innermost sheath, anandamaya kosha, which also gives us access to the dreaming samadhis, or savikalpas.

The center of our human embodiment remains in a deep sleep state in which, although not consciously, we go back to the divine source of our being. In deep sleep, we go back to our inner fire of consciousness where we purify and revitalize our energy and memory for another day. Nevertheless, the profound ignorance and the forgetfulness of Maya, the vision of the world, cover our knowledge of deep sleep.

When we fail to sleep properly, we are hardly conscious of our stay in deep sleep, so exhaustion and exhaustion will overtake all the rest we do. In the absence of good sleep, mind and prana, along with doshas, or biological humours, become imbalanced and induce the progressive breakdown of our organic structure. Starting with vata dosha, the central physiologic motivation power. Deep sleep balance our pranas and motivate us in our deeper wellbeing, without which our strength becomes unstable and depleted, which in Ayurvedic philosophy is called oyas. The immunity, stamina and resilience fail without deeper sleep, which eventually makes the body and mind collapse.

Deep sleep is known in Vedantic thinking as the muleavidia behind our lives, or' source ignorance.' It poses the main obstacle to every higher awareness. It is some form of darkness or ignorance that hides in us the greater reality of universal consciousness. But, if we learn to explore, understand and step beyond it, it is also the main path for consciousness liberation.

A yogi is seated on a spatially floating magic carpet that represents spiritual consciousness. The mountainous terrain below reflects the cinematic operation of the mind in waking and dreaming conditions. He resides in the unitive consciousness of the fourth state of Turiya profoundly in meditation.

Deep sleep is our natural samadhi, or a state of peace, but it comes from ignorance. The norm of it is tamasic. Nevertheless, it reflects the samadhi qualities of peace and happiness that can refresh the mind. Meditation cultivation of samadhi is a way to move back and forth deep sleep.

Until we learn to move beyond deep sleep through a deeper awareness, we will remain bound by karma, desire, birth and death. We will live in the shadow of darkness and unreality, which is our inability to see beyond the darkness of deep sleep into the inner light of truth. Deep sleep is not just a biological phenomenon; it is a spiritual limitation. It is the core mystery of our lives. Unless we learn to awaken from this primordial darkness, we will not know our true, cosmic reality.

The essence of our consciousness on this part in deep sleep is non-being, darkness and death. When we go through deep sleep into an ever-waking mind, the inner sun, the sun and life come up. By crossing deep sleep, crossing over death is not feasible. It is the alchemical path of the soul, which requires a transformation of our own core mind and identity.

Super consciousness, Turiya Avastha

Beyond these three more key and enigmatic ordinary states, the capacity for an ever-emerging consciousness does not endure every day fluctuations– the transcendent "fourth" or Turiya in yogical thought. This is the aim of higher yoga activities that take us beyond time and death. Turiya has the true secret, but we have to seek it with complete determination to uncover it. The state of common awareness underlies the other three states and transcends them.

Verse 7 of the Mandukya Upanishad explains this: "The one who is not conscious or unconscious, who is unseen, impalpable, indefinable, incomprehensible, unknown, whose very existence is that of an awareness of his own self, which absorbs all variety, is quiet and gentle; the fourth condition is what they refer to as the atman. It must be understood" (Vedic experience, p. 723). The fourth or ever waking condition is the samadhi's yogic state of consciousness or unity.

Those are three ever-changing wakeful, dream and deep-sleep states which can be expressed by Sri Swami Chidananda (1916-2008): "Because there is pure consciousness, non- consciously. Therefore, it is the Turiya Avastha– (fourth state), the eternal existence- consciousness concept which is Purusha– (the Supreme Being) that maintains and promotes a continually occurring and ever-changing trifle state or Avastha traya (three states of conscious mind: waking, dreaming, sleep). A clear and stable existence-consciousness or sat-chit serves all three countries. The conscious of life is super-consciousness "(in Swami, 1984, the Spiritual Life Trust Society, The Philosophy, Psychology, and Practice of Yoga). So, we can see that the life-consciousness-bliss of Advaita Vedanta (Satchidananda) is the absolute reality and the true state of consciousness.

This was also confirmed again in Adi Shankara's reflections on Mandukya Upanishad in the Encyclopaedia of Hinduism (India Heritage Research Foundation, 2010). "Turiya, or Brahman, is identical to the highest self. The truth is transcendent, non-dual, omnipresent, omniscient, everlasting, immutable, self-effulgent, restless, inexpressible, absolute and otologic.... Turiya has been defined as lieth beyond the three bodies and the five sheaths.... Thus, it is the non-dual state of mind, free of all the phenomenal predictions."

# Chapter Three

# Understanding Turiya

Advaita comprises three consciousness stages, namely waking (Jagrat), dreaming (Svapna), deep sleep (su fuckin') encountered Empirically by human beings, which correlate with the Three Bodies ' Theory.

The walking state is the first state, where we are aware of what's going around us in our daily world. This is the gross body.

The dreaming mind is the second state. This is the subtle body. The deep sleep is the third state. This is the causal body.

Advaita is also the fourth state of Turiya, which many of us describe as pure consciousness, that underlies the three conventional states of consciousness and transcends them. Turiya is the state of liberation where, according to the school of Advaita, the infinite (Ananta) and the non- different (Advaita) encounters the world in which ajativada (non-origination) has been captured, which is free from dualistic encounters. Candradhara Sarma said Sarma, the state of Turiya is the awareness that the basic Self is observable, without cause or effect, all consuming, without pain, joyful, unchanging, light-hearted, pure, immanent, and transcendent in everything. Those who have lived through the Turiya period have come to the pure consciousness of their own non-dual self as one with everything, truth, the truth, the well- known, the Jivanmukta for them.

In more ancient Sanskrit text, Advaita follows the basis of this ontological theory. Chapters 8.7 to 8.12 of Chandogya Upanishad speak, for example, about the' four states of consciousness' as alert, full of sleep, and deep sleep, and deeper sleep. In the Hindu scriptures one of the earliest mentions of Turiya is given in verse 5.14.3. In other early Upanishads the definition is discussed.

The early guru in the Advaita Vedanta was Gaudapada from around the 7th century. The grand guru of the great teacher, Adi Shankara's, is traditionally called one of the most important figures of Hindu philosophy. He is thought to be Shri Gaudapada's founder Charya Math, and Mandukya Kārika's author or compiler.

The Mandukya Kārika, also known as the Gaudapada Kārika, and the Agama Sastra, has also been written or compiled by Gaudapada. Gaudapada addresses in this work the topics of preconception, idealism, causality, truth and reality. The fourth state of silence (Turiya Avastha) is the same as that of AUM. It is the substratum of the three other nations. It is atyanta-shunyata, says Nakamura (total vacuity).

According to Comans, it's not possible to see how an unmistakable teaching of a permanent, underlying reality that was specifically referred to as "Self" could show early influence on Mahayana by the fourth realm. Michael Comans disputes that "the 4th (Catürtha) was perhaps inspired by the Sunyata of Mahayana Buddhism.".

The Comans also refer to Nakamura himself, who states later that the Vedantic philosophy inspired Mahayana sutras, such as the La fur-kāvatāra Sutra and the idea of Buddha-nature. Comans concluded that there can be no evidence that there is a trace of Buddhist philosophy in the lesson on the underlying Self, as the pre-Buddhist Brihadaranyaaka Upanishad can be traced back to this lesson.

Isaeva notes that in the teaching of the Buddhism texts and Mandukya Upanishad of Hinduism there are variations, since latter say that citta "consciousness" is similar to the atman "soul, self" of Upanishad, the eternal, unchangeable. Mandukya Upanishad and Gaudapada say the soul is there, while Buddhist schools say no soul or self exists.

Adi Shankara's

The three states of consciousness, namely waking (Jagrat), dreaming (Svapna), and deep sleep (susupti), that correspond to three bodies, have been outlined by Adi Shankara, based on the ideas advocated in the Mandukya Upanishad.

The first is an aware waking state in which we understand our everyday world. "External knowledge (Bahish-praynya), gross (sthula) and universal (vaishvanara) is established." That's the big body.

Second, the dreaming mind. The third one. "It is established as consciousness of the inside, subtle, (pravivikta, and burning)." That's the fragile body.

The third state is deep sleep. The basis of consciousness is undivided in this state. "The God of all things (Sarv-eshvar), the established of all, the inner power (anti-Yami), the origin and destruction of things created, (prabhav-apyayau hi bhutanam), the creator of all things created (yonyh sarvasya). This is the root cause.

There is a "I" (self-identity) and experience of the feelings in the awakening consciousness. There is no or no' I' in sleeping or dreaming; however, feelings and experience of thinking are present. Awakening and dreaming are not an absolute reality and spiritual a perception, as they have a dual existence of subject and subject, self, non-self, ego and non-ego.

The effect of these distracting is that we are guided by outside influences rather than internal awareness through confusion, desire and sorrow. We stay at our tumultuous surface and seldom come to the quiet depths of our being. In the thick, material world, we seek outer fulfilment and neglect the hidden happiness that resides in us.

The mystery of consciousness and its development is our lives. This is our key thing to learn. We ought to be driven to research our own minds carefully, not just the outside world. We will explore the profound consequences of the regular movements of our consciousness by waking and sleeping in the search of self-knowledge. In the Indian spiritual tradition such review was long established, as the pages before us indicate.

Dreams are often considered to be delusional, unreal and meaningless to everyday life. Yes, there's much more that we are told to dream and sleep in the west. Indian spiritual awareness gives an insight of dreams that can help us live a rich, more conscious life.

Kashmir Shaivism

The level is called turya is Kashmir Shaivism, the fourth world. There is no deep sleep or wakefulness. In reality, there is a crossroad between one of these three states: waking and dreaming, dreaming, deep sleep, deep sleep and waking. A fifth world of consciousness called Buryatia occurs in Cashmire's shaivism-the world outside Turiya. The state where one reaches liberation, otherwise known as Jivanmukta or Moksha, Turiya, also known as void or shunya is.

Will you know what the fourth mental state is? The human mind is a marvellous and amazing piece of complex machinery that can calculate quicker and better than a supercomputer. In particular, the different mental states that we encounter in order to understand consciousness properly should be known (turiya).

The human mind is divided into two main parts: Subconscious Mind

Conscious Mind

Conscious Mind is a logical part of our brain that regulates our consciousness or our thoughts at all times. This is the primary origin point of our daily choices, actions or reactions. This regulates our strength of will, long term memory, logical thought and critical thought.

The mind of thoughts is actually the consciousness at this time. You learn something on the outside and other mental functions on the inside.

Subconscious Mind is the' deeper' part of the mind that has to deal with thousands of things at all times and store anything with different degree of meaning in our lives. It's a kind of' auto pilot' that operates without even realizing it. It is similar to a computer's hard disk that stores information from other computer / mind bits. It's responsible for managing our thoughts, feelings, behaviours, principles, defensive responses, creativity, intuition and some of the memory in our minds. (Some researchers also discuss the' unconscious mind' which normally regulates the physical processes.)

The are 4 predominant Brainwave States or Frequencies at which the mind operates

Digital EEG Machine

Such specific disorders are graded from one neurological point to another at any given moment according to the intensity of the prevailing brainwave signals. The intensity and frequency of' Hertz' was measured by means of an electrocardiogram (EEG).

Beta: This is where our mind normally works in our everyday lives. In this climate, we are conscious of everything around us and pay little attention. Typically, only one side of our brain works at this stage. Beta becomes usually characterized by brainwave cycles 15-40 Hz (cycles per second) higher Beta frequency cycles, which typically correlate tension, anxiety or' over thinking,' as the mind is confused or negatively reacts to a given situation. Both hypertension, heart rates, blood flow increases, cortisone production, and glucose intake are high brain waving beta frequency. In general, if you're worried about your health, you don't want to experience high beta too often. (For certain methods, this is not listed below)

Alpha: Sweet relaxation or a mild daydream. If you are driving a car and just cruising around or get caught up in a good book you can be example of a situation in Alpha and a sort of losing course in which you are happening. Meditation is generally done in alpha frequencies to oscillate brain waves. During intervals between 9Hz and 14Hz the brain works. Alpha is usually seen as a combination of partial consciousness and partial predominance of the subconscious. If your brain is alpha-frequently, it is useful to absorb information and is considered highly desirable for effective study and concentration. Alpha makes use of the left part of the brain for processing.

Theta: A profound rest where the conscious mind ' switches off' for the most part, and the subconscious mind flourishes and wanders through its own medium. Sleep, dreaming, very deep stimulation is usually the main aim of many hypnotists and helps their customers get to their goals. Theta shows a 5hz to 8hz brainwave range. Theta, where thoughts, images and suggestions are more likely to enter the subconscious mind and we are aware less of what is happening around us.

Delta: Really very deep relaxation / sleep in motion with full subconscious mind. Delta is known and desirable in the depths of sleep, because the physical body starts to recover and heal in this state at an increased level. If you are in an advanced state of meditation, you may be in a waking delta state. This state is related to the experience of kundalini. Slow brain waves at 1Hz–4Hz are known as Delta. Ironically, a highly qualified Hypnotist who is capable of taking a client through Delta is able to perform such a process by using hypnosis as a substitute for anaesthesia during various medical procedures.

Transitioning Between the Different States

As the human mind shifts spontaneously according to the current conditions, situations, individuals or occurrences of the person between the different mind-states. You will stimulate the brain to various levels artificially. As an extreme example, we often get into a coma when we are involved in a serious accident or injury. This is the way the brain will react in an emergency to reach the deepest realms of the delta immediately for increased physical healing, trauma safety and mental regeneration. It is an excellent example of the normal brain reaction to a situation in which brainwave activity for instinctual defence is lowered.

For both social and sometimes wrong intentions, we may deliberately cause a shift in our attitude. Stage hypnotists also call on theta for the amusement of a sudden shift of the brainwave frequency by a rapid hypnotic induction. Although many people find this funny and the power of hypnosis is illustrated, the other way around is not to laugh. There are several examples of the reckless use of these mass manipulation techniques, which can actually be a devastating use for positive change.

A person is invited to function in several brain wave Frequency States artificially. There are many types. These include hypnosis, meditation, sound and music, relaxation, food, alcohol,

yoga, Pilates, video games, Television, driving, reading, etc. When you learn the best way of decreasing your mental state to Alpha, Theta and Delta, you can have many emotional, financial, and physical positive benefits. Of example, hypnosis is good to place you in theta, then use direct instructions, which your unconscious mind will then accept, of positive and lasting changes in your mind and body.

Meditation is also beneficial for preserving a light alpha state, in which information and input can be consciously interpreted to change the emotions and feelings. Audio and audio like the binaural beats, white noise, theta rhythm and other sluggish, repeating sounds of the trance can help you overcome insomnia and better sleep, conduct self-meditation, auto-hypnosis and deep relaxation on the alpha, theta, and in the delta. Deep relaxation is known to help the mind and the body reliably every day! This promotes clarity of thought, focus and improved good health and a healthy mind, body and emotion.

The fourth state of mind is close to the achievement of God or super awareness. In a greatly ancient philosophical novel, True experience of the self is you being aware of who you really are'."

When a snake discards his worn-out skin and then doesn't know about it, a human likewise doesn't know what his body becomes. If body consciousness does not conceive of this earthly life, suffering and joy, freedom and slavery, etc., disappear and his mind enters the 4th state. When the practitioner goes beyond that level, he becomes Brahman (god) himself, and by the enigmatic words "No, that's not" the Upanishads identify this level. Brahman has nothing to say.

What is Turiya – The Fourth State of Mind

God is said to be omnipresent. God exists in every part of your body. This means God exists. Science assumes that the body contains millions of cells, and everyone has intelligence. Turiya is the context to which the three different states of consciousness are subjected and transcended. The states of consciousness are: arousing consciousness, dreaming, and dreamless sleekness. In the Hindu philosophy, Turiya is a simple awareness, chaturtha, paramahmsa.

The state above deep, dreamless sleep that activates the superconscious. Turiya is the fourth state of consciousness in which each man rests in Satchidananda ("eternal, eternally aware and ever fresh bliss"), Swami Sivananda says. The person has reached the final release from the ego-awareness and is united with the infinite spirit. Turiya refers both to Atman and to Brahman, the eternal self, who represent their divine union.

The single soul understands the three waking, dreaming and sleeping states in Turiya and transcends them. He moves beyond Brahman's gross presence in the material world, Brahman's subtle dimension in the dream World, and deep sleep induces the infinite form. As a pure knowledge and joy, he knows its true nature. Therefore, in the outer world he is saved from desire, delusion and duality.

Turiya is not a State other than the bigger states, but as super consciousness penetrates all layers of reality. Ramana Maharishi considers Turiya to be the only truth as the natural state which permeates the other Ones. The Mandukya Upanishad talks of Turiya as a pure consciousness that the mind can not explain, can not understand and can not be understood, but eventually realized as the one true self.

The Four Levels of Consciousness

It implies that God's power is concentrated in every cell of the body. But it's resting. In the body lie resting both gods and goddesses. You don't meditate because you don't. You just feed, drink, procreate and say lies in your consciousness. The only thing that is probable is jagrita, swapna and sushupti. Only these three consciousness states are known to you. You are up, or you dream, or you fall asleep. You're not aware of a fourth condition. But a human being called Turiya, which is a higher consciousness, is a fourth state of consciousness. The practice of one-pointiness of the mind will achieve this higher consciousness. Turiya is the history behind the three rising states of consciousness and transcends them. The states of consciousness are: waking, dreaming and sleepless.

The Mandukya Upanishad's Turiya is addressed in verse 7. But in the oldest Upanishads the term is included. For example, the "four states of consciousness" are addressed as alive, filled with sleep, deep sleep and beyond deep sleep, as in chapters 8.7 through 8.12 of Changoya- Upanishad. Similarly, in Chapter 5.14, Brihadaranyaka Upanishad talks about the state of Turiya. Maitri Upanishad addresses in Sections 6.19 and 7.11 the fourth state(turiya).

As you gradually ascend over the three states of Jagrita, Swapna, and Sushupti, a fourth state is created during dhyana and a new sky, your consciousness wakes. TURIYA or the Fourth State is a state where each soul rests in its very Sat-Chit-Ananda Svarupa, in the Nirvikalpa Samadhi.

You may follow these five principle practices to achieve this fourth state (Turiya).:

Imagine you've been dreaming. You bought a plot in that sight and build a house. The house is done and the house warming ceremony you deem your dear friends. But in the centre, because of some thing, you were awake from your sleep. Nevertheless, the sight goes on. You send your friends a sumptuous dining and plan the party together with a great host service. But because you're out of your dream, you won't be aware of these things. Only think of the whole world as a dream for a moment. Now you are awoken again, for instance, in the centre.

You have no idea what is happening in the world out of the dream now. As nobody is seeing the planet, now after you wake up, you won't know or remember what's going on or was going on here. These ideas give a different kind of mind calm and spiritual joy.

In the same way, what if we assume that our mind is just like a puzzle and a reflection on pure consciousness is inside it? You might know the concept of mirage in a desert? All mind and ego are not real things, but are superimposed on pure consciousness (as is the mirage on the rays of the sun). These reflections are useful to erase our ego.

The practitioner should always believe that he is about 10-20 feet away from his body. He needs only to believe he's a body's witness. In this condition, the practitioner has no body pain or enjoyment, respect, dishonour etc. In times of even greatest and most extreme suffering and tragedy, his mind remains calm and peaceful. He is truly peaceful.

The Waker who experiences the gross physical world is the first quarter.

The second quarter is the one who experiences the subtle mind-projected world, he is also called the dreamer

The third quarter is the one who experiences the unmanifest world, he is also called the deep sleeper

The fourth quarter, also called Turiya, is Atman itself, which encounters itself. The world is completely absent in this state. The world does not exist, together with the body, mind and intellect. Anything other than Atman is completely non-existent.

Therefore, the fourth state is indicated with the aid of the three States. The three countries are like AUM's three letters and the fourth the silence.

Silence lies in AUM, but no AUM in the deep silence. Silence is overlaid by the AUM, but there is also silence without the AUM. Similarly, Turiya is superimposed on the three states of waking, dreaming and deep sleep, but Turiya has no countries. It is pure undifferentiated universal mass of the Beatitude of Existence.

This is the state of illumination. A person is free of all misconceptions after he has reached this condition. The once accepted world loses all its sense of reality. It is regarded as an illusion without any basis.

Just as you return after sleep, you can return to a wakeful condition after you are in Turiya. Jiwan Mukta is the one who witnessed the Turiya. Whilst there is a consciousness of the world for a realized human, its illusionary nature remains uncertain. There is therefore no association with the world and no association with the body, mind and spirit. He sees the world as a picture. The Atman alone is real to him.

Just as you recall and think about the state of sleep. The Jiwan Mukta is in the state of Turiya and speaks in sacred language.

Turiya

Imagine now if you are in front of a hill. The ages pass here, and there is corn in their eyes. with great enthusiasm. They touch at every moment and yet they can not cross a small stream of water.

Anthill

These behaviours are considered to be dumb as you're not an ant. Attempt to be a superman and look at this world in the same way. Then you will know that the world of ants is childish like every beauty, money, riches, cities, etc. Becoming a spiritual soul, the mind is now. You shall always enjoy Divine Joy

Think powerfully that all activities in this world are led and controlled by the God Almighty. You will be disappointed by this practicing of spirituality. There is nothing, but you look at him and his symbols. You must think that your life and actions are also governed by him, as you are a small part of the Universe. Your lives are dominated by His will. Faith is critical in this reasoning. This is not a fatalism but a fact. You need to be convinced that the only thing you can do is to raise your hands and not your own. In the advanced phase of this spiritual practice, the sense of self is totally annihilated and the practitioner is persuaded that his will governs the actions of this world and his body. You'll start to think you're a marionette under Almighty God's influence. Your life will become holy, peaceful and glorious under his guidance. Such spiritual rituals should not be practiced like other meditations in one place and at a certain time.

You have to revolve in your mind all day long the above thoughts. You should eventually realize that this theory is just the Almighty's sport. Any frustration, frustration, embarrassment, etc. that he could be exposed to will he take seriously. Spiritual practice 5 is supreme among all the above five spiritual practices and brings quick results in the fourth state (Turiya).

The Atman is recorded to be four quarters in Mandukya Upanishad. It is planned to have four quarters in order to teach the seekers. There are no divisions in Atman by themselves. It's like the one Rupee Coin, covered in four quarters but only one whole coin.

A spiritual journey

The trip is always incomplete, as it never begins. People often start the journey of spirituality with the discovery of religion. Some of them lose their faith & go on to therapy.

What is spirituality, however? The concept ' spirituality is the' Being OF THE SPIRIT.' Do you feel the spirit being??

What are the spirit's qualities? There are many people who try to explain it, it's shapeless, ageless, no start, no end, there are many names– jiva atma, param atma. Many people would say it's in and some will lead you to find it. Many people would say that Zen is the way, others will teach you mantras. Many things get complicated by meanings & phrases. The paradox is that I only hear words that are not to be explained. Some may think of God as THE SPIRIT and then give GOD qualities– Babies, Compassions, etc.

It is, it is reality that is just the representation of humanity that we want to see in Heaven. Heaven isn't just the creator, the life-giver, but also the death giver, the life-giver. If nothing is outside the Lord, gladness and happiness are as much a part of God as sorrow and pain.

But it is the little spirit of humanity that seeks happiness and therefore the blessing of goodness, wealth and peace. Neither can anyone ever dare to ask for pain or trouble. But if you really want to be closer to God, it is not that you consider God the most in times of difficulty?

So, what more do you want– sensational pleasure and harmony, or Heaven!!! The road away from GOD is even the search of illumination!!!

DIRECT???? –It's the truth, however!

Are you looking for God or illumination? Which one is better than that? Some might say, a tricky question because the achievement of enlightenment is not God's goal? NO. It's not that way. The search for knowledge often leads to a "GURU" — explained just by a master who dispel the darkness of ignorance by the truth / light of knowledge.

If, then, light dissipates obscurity. What's darkness, how do light know? Since there is no darkness in his presence. So, if God is, how can ignorance come about? Ignorance is dispelled by the very embrace of God. The way to be illuminated is thus easy. Be in GOD's presence!!

And GOD is not there to punish one contrary to other religious beliefs. It is literally the consequence of one's own karmas, both positive and negative, that one must undergo. It contributes to karma for every thought and action. What's the result then??

"Faith– QUALITY" is the way out. The norm of the spirit must be embraced. You have to look at instance to comprehend the spirit. Everybody is treated equally by law. The deer consuming the lion, even succeeding in human life or natural death, are all born, and their grazing is eaten. Therefore, by nature, birth & death is a natural process. Always at work, new fresh emerges. But intellect but physical shape change as part of the evolutionary process.

However, in order to understand the mechanism, the process of conception– merging an egg & sperm into one intelligent cell– can be understood. And a full child comes from that one cell – head, arms, legs, etc. One cell's knowledge extends across a whole body. Likewise, the process of universe creation. The whole universe has evolved from one cell. The essence of "SPIRIT QUALITY" lies within. Human Being.

At the same time, several cells are formed and each of them has the intellect to develop into their normal state– a lion, a wolf, a human body or a plant. Each cell is flourishing into its existence.

It's not the whole or the whole. It's normal. It's normal. It's not that. Each cell of its different nature grows. And total relaxation. You're not pretending to be someone else. The wolf is not a horse, or the rose is not a lotus. We are all familiar and their natural environment.

This is representative of the Sanskrit word "SAHAJA." Of course, you are comfortable with yourself and who you are. It's stress-creating to try and be what you're not. Be natural. Be natural. With yourself comfortable. You are what you are, for nature has created you in this way.

This does not mean that you are relinquishing every effort. For the process of nature and natural instincts, efforts are important. For example, you need to make efforts to have this meal if you're hungry. A woman has to find grass, the tiger has to capture the hunt, the farmer has to work on heritage and in modern society, everybody does what is done to acquire the paper or electronic money and to buy food. You have to go to the restaurant or pick up the phone and order in, even if you are ready to use. You'll be praised for your contributions and be commensurate with your contributions. However, if you make efforts, you will get good karma, even for a good cause. And then you will acquire the fruit of this karma, which you call a better life. Until this time is coming, all the world's attractions will not be enticing enough.

And then you're searching for more. You launch a quest then. And this quest also leads you around the town. Although everything you need to do is remain silent. You'll find what you need if you're there. Discover yourself. Discover your natural self.

And this is a straightforward process. Be natural!! Be natural!! You don't have to travel throughout the earth or the cosmos. It is in you, the world. There was only one cell that had the wisdom to develop into the entire body. You have the wisdom in you and the secret you are looking for lies inside you.

Enjoy indoors! And if you are the beginning of yourself, you can only discover yourself in you. Be sahaja. Be sahaja. Be natural. Be natural. Wake up to your "QUALITY-SPIRIT." Be comfortable with who you are. And you're going to find out "WHO YOU ARE!!"

The condition in which the soul is sensitive to the vibration, touch, and other gross artifacts by means of the energies of the sun and of the other gods and through the instrumentality of those quatorze: spirit, intellect, consciousness, ego and the ten sense organ. Once the living being is sensitive to sound, touch, and other significant artifacts –even in the absence of the latter –by reason of the unfulfilled waking desire, it is called the soul's dreaming condition.

The Eastern Mind distinguishes consciousness into two states: one when we are awake or the first; the second when we dream; the third, when we sleep deep, when we have dreams; and the fourth after all three. What do we call this awake state of mind?? In two ways information can be achieved: mediate and immediate. Mediate understanding medium knowledge in certain cases, not directly, implicitly. Senses are the medium, the doors by which the extension beyond us is understood. But the information gained is indirect; The mediator is in between, not a face-to-face experience. The senses are mediators and it is not a simple knowledge, nor an understanding, when senses inform us about something. The senses are not just passive listeners, they are also active translators; they enforce it, add to the knowledge.

So, when the senses inform the consciousness of something it's not a passive receptiveness; the senses have attached something to it, perceived it, put something on it. This interference makes every consciousness an illusory reality, and every person begins to live in his own mind. The MAYA, the madness, says this world, the ancient east mind. That's not the real, the goal: it's something that you made. Each is in his own world, and so many worlds as minds exist. If two people are together, there's a collision between two worlds. And otherwise, if you didn't know the goal as it was.

The second dimension, the alternate level of knowledge of the world, is not by sight, but by emotions. Yet human consciousness can be clearly met: sight is lost, yet awareness still exists. Such information is about the facts, as no mediator was present. You knew it straight away now. Knowing the truth by the emotions is Maya; knowing the truth straight away, face to face is BRAHMAN's. Everything we know appears to be the same, but the KNOWER shifts. If you use senses, you create an illusionary perception; if you don't use the words, then you face the reality.

Meditation is the way to drop the senses, drop the windows and be with nothing in reality. The Rishi says that the first consciousness, the awake state of mind, JAGRUT, is this contact with the world through the senses. When through the senses you come into contact with the world, it is jagrut– the awake mind of your mind.

The second state, deeper than the wake-up state, is dreaming. Dreaming is a secondary, albeit deeper, replacement state. Whatever was left unfulfilled when you were awake must be done. Brain is inclined to finish things. You can not create a dream if you leave it incomplete. The mind usually finishes something. There's something restless inside, you cannot complete it. You saw a lovely figure, but you couldn't look at it as you liked. There will now be a continuing incompletion. You should inhibit it when you're awake– you're busy and the suppression is necessary. But when you sleep it unfolds a dream and completes the thing While you sleep.

The rishi says that this state of dream means without the senses ' instrumentality. The senses are locked-they don't know the world around you. You are now in your cells, in your body, but you can still create your own worlds. It becomes possible to make your own worlds in dreams because your mind shaped what you learned and thought, everything was stored in it. It is an accumulation not only in this life, but also in all the lives that one has lived; not only in human life but also in animal life; but also, in animal life.

You can become a tree in a dream and a lion in a fantasy. You were once a tree: there is a memory, it can unfold. This unfolding of past recollections, past lives just means that you have never completely, just partially, lived. You didn't love fully, you didn't feel utterly furious, you weren't totally Everything. It's everything left. There are so many incomplete items within, which establish the situation of dreaming. When you start living completely, it's all over, dreams stop.

Since he left no aspect missing, a Christ, a buddha, will not dream. This moment is necessary, says Jesus, live it entirely. Don't remember the next moment; don't worry about the other moment you've left. The ones that have gone are not, and those that are not yet here, have not yet arrived. They are both non-existential. The only existential time is this moment, this very moment, this passive moment. Live there! Stay there! And just set everything else aside. Be absolutely in it, then no dream, then it's all over. And by night nothing is incomplete and needs to be done as you fall into sleep. And when dreaming ceases, the mind is more awake.

It's the second state: to dream. When you stop dreaming, you get more wake; when you don't dream in the night, and when you get awake in the morning you have fresher, more alive, more innocent eyes. There is no dust in your eyes, no smoke; without smoke, the flame is visible. Dreaming makes your eyes smoke. And someone who dreams at night, still continues to dream at daytime. A continuous dream film is always up deep down. You hear me: just close your eyes and look inside and a vision emerges. You are too busy outside, so you can't watch your inner dreams; but the dreaming is still going on.

See heaven; no stars are here. Where did they go? Where did they go? They can't go anywhere; they're there in the dark, but we can't see them only due to the heat. Our eyes are so occupied with the light that they can't enter it. They are still there. They're still there. You can even look at the stars when you can fall into a deep well during the day, because then the night is broken and stars appear again. You always dream just like that. If you are engaged in the outer world, however, the vision continues inside without your attention. As soon as you aren't busy, relax, you remember the vision. This is an ongoing- indeed a continuous- state. And this dream is more symbolic than anything we call awake about your mind, because it is less constrained, less suppressed, exposed and therefore more real.

So, if you can know your dreams, if you can know your dreams, you are known for much. You can't deceive — at least in dreams. You are not part of your will yet; you are not ready. This is why you're and wild, so animal like, you're not the master. It must be penetrated only transcended in this second stage. And then will we hit third –deeper still, deep sleep, amazing night.

The deeper you go, the closer you get to be. The larger the core is, the closer the world is to the centre. Such three circles are cantered in the middle: awake, dreaming and sleeping. These are three spheres of focus. If you overcome all three of them, you're instantly face to face. Then you center yourself there. The emphasis is all about it.

The objective is to hit the dead. This emphasis should be deep within the center of the universe. This attention is God's realization.

You must stop dreaming, you must stop dreaming. Dream must be solved– the obstacle is dreaming. The reality can never be understood by a dreaming mind, a dreaming mind must exist in an illusionary way. The problem is dreaming, and if it starts dreaming... It stops when desire ends, when you want to stop, when you start living moment by moment, here and now. When two words "here" and "now" can be recalled, it ceases to dream. Be here and there, and you can't dream, because dreaming still comes from the past and the future. It comes from the past; it goes into the future.

In the moment, dreaming can't be. It is difficult to be in the moment and to dream; they never meet. So, if you're awake, aware, attentive to the time here and now, dream ends. And when it's time to dream, you can become alive, truly conscious. This consciousness will reach the third state of consciousness when you are awake: dreamless sleep. There is really a term for it– SUSHUPTI, in no other language than Hindi. There's no word– sushupti– in any language.

Sleep doesn't become sushupti, so we have to give sleep to the DREAMLESS. It's not just sleeps; it's sleepless — no wave of the night, no waves of the vision. The sea is completely silent, there is no night to trouble. Then you are in sushupti– a third state, unpopular sleep, unpopular sleep. But you can not know it unless you stop dreaming. You can only get to know the deep, and otherwise you will only know the waves. The waves will pause. Waves are on the shore, so you see the waves, not the deep, when you see them. The waves have to stop altogether. Only then can the ocean, the wave less ocean– dreamless sleep become conscious of it for the first time. And if you can know sleep without dreaming, you surpass sleep. Only when you are conscious of it transcends sleep. And then you are the fourth turiya; then all three have passed through.

The quest is this fourth thing; the search is this fourth. It is critical for this fourth effort. And you can continue to dream and dream and dream– this fourth state can never be reached by dreaming. That is why the desireless, non-ambitious insistence is so intense. The buddhas continue to say, (Do not want to), because dreaming can not stop if you want to. The buddhas continue to say, "Don't be bound," because the dream can not be stopped if you are bound. Don't be greedy, don't wait, don't think about the future, because you can't stop dreaming. And you will never be until dreaming ceases. Never can you be! You will always become just a turn:' a' becomes' b' because' b' becomes' c,'' c' transforms into' d'– and always the search for the screen. Instead you continue running and never come; instead you continue to become that and that and you never are a person.

The creature is here. Drop your dreams and you have always been there, but you never knew. All meditation techniques are anti-dream efforts, only devices that negate dreams.

Three phases must be observed by New Morning Meditation– Dynamic Meditation. They should be pursued with the full vigour. You have to do everything– nothing less is going to do. The first move is to respire quickly. Respire as quickly as possible as we use breathing as a weapon. It must be an inner hammering to unwrap the sprayed electricity. Therefore, use the serpent as a hammer to wake it up. Don't retain; totally give in. I will continue to encourage you for 10 minutes to make every effort. Everything you can do at your height, your climax.

You must be in a catharsis in the second step. Dance, run, scream, laugh-but do something, whatever happens to you. It requires effort– everything inside has to be flung outwards. This catharsis leads to a pure and profound purification.

You need to use' hoo' in the third step! "So, continue to cry," shit! Hoo! Hoo! Hoo! Huh! Huh! "It is also a hammer to be used. This mantra," hoo, "goes down into the MULADHAR, into the sex center, and brings up the energy. After thirty minutes, step four— we'll lie, as if dead, waiting for the divine to come down. Make yourself a place so that you can be totally mad. Create space for you. Don't be within a group. Don't be within a crowd.

Close the blindfold to your eyes now. Make room for it. Look and see, you're going to jump and dance and get completely mad.

# Chapter Four

# The Upanishad

The Upanishads are ancient Sanskrit teaching texts and Hindu beliefs, mostly followed by religious traditions such as Buddhism and Jainism. It is one of the oldest writings in the Hindu, the Vedas, which deal with meditation, philosophy and spiritual knowledge; other parts of the Vedas deal with mantras, blessings, rituals, ceremonies and sacrifices Of ancient times the Upanishads played an important part in the development of spiritual ideas in one of the main literatures in the history of Indian religions and culture.. The Upanishads alone are widely recognized of all Vedic literature and their main concepts are at the spiritual heart of Hinduism.

Currently the Upanishads are called Vedanta. The concept of Vedanta as "last chapters, parts of the Veda" and as "Subject, the highest aim of the Veda." These are the central ideas in all Upanishads and the center of the philosophy of Brahman (the last reality) and Tetman (the mind, the self). They are their thematic matter. Two prominent monistic schools of Hinduism are established along with the Bhagavad Gita and the Brahmasutra, the mukhya Upanishads (known collectively as Prasthanatrayi).

There are more than 200 Upanishads known, about the first dozen are the oldest and most significant, and the main

Upanishads (mukhya). The mukhya Upanishads are found mostly in the latter part of the Brahmanas and Aranyakas and have been recalled and transmitted orally for centuries by each generation. The early Upanishads were pre-Common Period, of which five were possibly pre-Buddhist (6th century BC), ranging from 322 to 185 BC into Maurya. Of the others, 95 Upanishads are part of the canon of Muktika from the last century to about the fifteenth century A.C. New Upanishads were still written in the early modern and modern period after 108 in the Muktika canon but were mostly concerned with subjects not related to the Vedas.

In the early 19th century they have began to attract attention from a west audience with the Upanishads ' translation. The Upanishads influenced Arthur Schopenhauer profoundly, calling it "the development of the highest human knowledge." The philosophical aspects of the Upanisads and major Western thinkers were discussed in the modern era.

The term Upani Tad in Sanskrit (from up to "up" and "neither" to "sit") means that the student is sitting next to the teacher and gaining spiritual knowledge. Many examples of the dictionary include "esoteric idea" and "secret guidance." Monier-Williams ' Sanskrit Notes: "The Upanishad means to show the supreme spirit's knowledge and put a stop to ignorance."

In his comments on the Ka Subha and the Brihadarenyak Upanishad, Adi Shankaracharya explains that the term means "knowledge of oneself;" that is "knowledge of oneself" or "knowledge of Brahma." The word is written in several Upanishads ' chapters, such as the fourth verse in the 13th volume in Chandogya Upanishad's first book. In these lines, Robert Hume translates the term Upanishad as "hidden doctrine," as does Paul Deussen, and Patrick Olivelle, as "hidden relations," as "mystical sense."".

Understanding and being are the same thing. Being is the only way to understand. And there are two development dimensions: consciousness and life. More and more, you will learn and remain the same. BE more. Be more. BE more. The being has to grow; not awareness, not learned information-but it has to grow. There must be more knowledge, not knowledge. And only spiritual development is of consciousness. Anything but a burden that adds to your knowledge.

It's always dangerous to play with the realities, because they are going to destroy you. You are going to be born again. We have only been pregnant for years, life so life and not the conception. We are only pregnant, we are only a seed, because nobody is prepared to pay the price. And before you come to our searching joy, you have a deep misery to go through. This is a deep pain. You can't escape the pain of conception.

With the ego, you're never free. All errors are born from the ego. Therefore, thinking that you are being rescued already means that you are still vulnerable. The more we learn, the less it is. The more we learn. The other shore is not just the unknown but the unknown. This is the mystery. It is this kind of intelligence that makes that mystical. This is mystery: you know and still don't know.

Like blood in the body, money is still circulating. Information cannot be transferred like money; it is impossible to transfer the information. So, what should I do? What should the disciple do to the master? "Give us strength," the master prays. We should aspire together; we should aspire together, "but we shoot straight for TOGETHER. The master's family– a family member because they're not teachers.

The correct enquiry starts with prayer; the enquiry is not real, otherwise. Doubt is only a illness without prayer. Doubt becomes only the form of inquiring and questioning with a prayerful mood and a priestly spirit. Ambiguity is perfect if there's trust inside. A positive sign is a real doubt. The lack of trust remains; doubt is only a tool. There can be no ambiguity. When ambiguity is the lack, then it's a never-ending retreat: you will start to doubt and doubt and doubt and there's no end to it. You continue to fall into greater indecisiveness, with doubt. Doubt must not be the goal to meet anywhere. Use it as a tool– it's beneficial, but keep your mind focused on faith. Doubt disappears.

There's a chance –you're gone. Doubt is therefore a self-destructive process; it's suicidal, for you are demanding and not open to receiving. You are not ready for the reply, but you inquire. You continue to ask and miss the answer to your question.

Prayer means welcome, celebrations– you are safe. You are responsive. Be available, ask, be free and ask. This UPANISHAD begins with the prayer, the enquiry and then the questioning of the God Force to help. Curiosity is not only about prayer challenging. It becomes a genuine quest with prayer.

Muktika canon: major and minor Upanishads

Over 200 Upanishads are known, of which one, the Muktika Upanishad, was built up in 1656 and includes a list of 108 Canonical Upanishads. These were further split into Upanishad, aligned with shakti, sannyas, shaivism (the god Shiva), yoga and sāmānya (general and sometimes referred to as Sāmānya-Vedanta), and shaivism (the god Vishnua). These are also divided into the Shaktish.

Some Upanishads are called "sectarian" because they pose their ideas by a particular god or goddess of a different Hindu tradition, like Vishnu, Shiva, Shakti or a combination of those, like the Upanishad of Skanda. Such traditions tried to connect their Vedic texts, thus affirming the Upanishad, Čruti, in their language. Much of these secular Upanishads, for instance the Rudrahridaya Upanishad and the Mahanarayana Upanishad, contend that all the Hindu gods and goddesses are the same, that they are an all-embracing feature and manifestation of Brahman.

Mukhya Upanishads

It is possible to split the Mukhya Upanishads into sections. Brihadaranyaka and Chandogya, the oldest, are among the early ages.

Early in the middle of the 1th century BCE, the Aitareya, Kau Fastidieni and Taittiriya Upanishads date from around the 4th to 1st centuries BCE, approximately corresponding with earliest Sanskrit epics. There is a chronology suggesting that after the 5th century BC Aitareya, Taittiriya, Kausitaki, Mundaka, Prasna, Katha Upanishads had an influence on the Buddha; another suggestion challenges the assumption and dates it regardless of the date of birth of buddha. Following these major Upanishads, Kena, Mandukya and Isa Upanishads are generally placed, but these are other scholars. There is little knowledge of the writers except those mentioned in the texts, such as Yajnavalkayva and Uddalaka. Occasionally, a number of women are also present, such as Gargi and Maitreyi, Yajnavalkayva's aunt.

Each of the major Upanishads may be affiliated with one of the four Vedas (shakhas) exegesis colleges. Several Shakhas, of which only a few remain, are said to exist. The modern Upanishads often have little connection to the Vedic corpus and have not been mentioned or commented upon by any great Vedanta philosopher: their language varies from that of the classical Upanishads, being less descriptive and more formalized. As a result, they are not difficult for the average reader to understand.

New Upanishads

The Upanishads have not been classified as recent ones, but have been discovered and written beyond the Muktika anthology of 108 Upanishads. In 1908, for example, Friedrich Schraders, who attributed it to the first Upanishad prose, revealed four previously unknown Upanishads in newly found manuscripts called Bashkala, Chhagaleya, Arsheya and Saunaka. The text of three of them was incomplete and incomplete, probably poorly preserved or corrupted, namely the Chhagaleya, Arsheya and Saunaka.

Ancient Upanishads have long been respected for Hindu tradition and writers of different sectarian texts have sought, by calling their texts Upanishads, to benefit from this reputation. Such hundreds of "new Upanishads" cover various topics from biology to rejection of sectarian theory. It consisted of the early modern era (~1600 CE) from the last decades of the first millennium BC. Although more than two dozen minor Upanishads date back to the previous 3.00 CE, many of these new texts with the title "Upanishad" came into being during the first half of the 2nd millennium CE. For example, the main Shakta Upanishads specifically discuss doctrinal and interpretative differences between the two main Tantric sects of a major shakticism known as Shri Vidya upasana. The many lists available for the authentic Shakta Upani Godads differ, representing the sect of their compilers, to prevent them from providing proof that they "locate" in the tantric tradition. The content of tantric texts weakens even their status as a Upani lifestyle. Sectarian texts like these are not considered shruti and thus the authority of the modern Upanishads is not recognized as a scripture in Hinduism.

The four Vedas– Rigvida, Samaveda, Yajurveda (the two main versions or Yajurveda Samhitas– are Shukla Yajurveda, Krishna Yajurveda, and Atharvaveda) all are related to Upanishads. During the modern era, the ancient Upanishads that were rooted in texts in the Vedas were removed from the Vedic layers of Brahman and Aranyaka, compiled into distinct texts and collected in Upanishads anthology. The lists are related to one of the four Upanishads and are many of them, and in all of India these lists are inconsistent with the Upanishads and the manner in which the newer Upanishads are supposedly assigned to the old Vedas. The list collected in South India was made the most popular by the 19th century based on Muktika Upanishad, and was written in Telugu. The 52 Upanishads were most famous in northern India.

The list of Muktika Upanishads contains 108 Upanishads the first thirteen as Mukhayas, twenty like Sāmānya Vedanta, ten like Sannyasa, fourteen like Vaishnava, twelve as Shaiva and eight as Shakta. Two as Yoga. The following table shows 108 Upanishads recorded in the Muktika. The most important and outstanding mukhya Upanishads are.

A plurality of worldviews characterized the Upanishadic era. While some Upanishads are considered to be' monitory,' others are dualist, including the Katha Upanishad. In comparison to the non-dualistic Upanishads at the base of its Vedanta school, Maitri is one of the Upanishads who tend toward dualism that form the classical Samkhya and the Yoga School of Hinduism. We have a variety of ideas.

The Upanishads have inspired Indian thought as well as faith and life since their conception, says Sarvepalli Radhakrishnan. Only because they were discovered (Shruti) are respected by the Upanishads, but because they provide compelling philosophical ideas. The Upanishads are treaties of Brahmanism that is facts of the absolute hidden truth. "It is a strictly personal effort to reach the facts" their analysis of philosophy presumes. Word is a road to liberation in the Upanishads, Radhakrishnan says, and pursuit of knowledge by way of life is the philosophy.

The Upanishads includes metaphysical theory sections which were at the heart of Indian traditions. Chandogya Upanishad, for instance, contains one of Ahimsa's (non-violence) earliest known concepts of ethics. In the most ancient Upanisads and a large number of later Upanishads are also discussion of other ethical principles such as Damah (temperance) and self-restraint, Satya (truthfulness), Dāna (charity). The Brihadaranyaka Upanishad, the oldest Upanishad is stated likewise in the Karma doctrine.

Development of thought

Though rituals are underlined by the hymns of the Vedas and liturgical manuals are used by the Brahmas for these Vedic rituals, the Upanishad Spirit fundamentally opposes rituals. The older Upanishads also incorporated more and more violent ritual assaults. Everyone who adores a divinity other than themselves, in the Upanishad Brihadaranyaka, is considered a domestic animal of the gods. Those who indulge themselves in acts of sacrifice are paroled by the Upanishad Chandogya in a procession of dogs singing Om! Let's just sleep. Let's recover. God!

-Om! Drink it Let's.

Kaushitaki Upanishad states that "the ritual of introspection" must be replaced by "external rituals such as Agnihotram offered in the morning and evening, and that" not rituals but knowledge should be the solicitude. "Mundaka Upanishad explains how people have been called upon, given rewards, terrified and deceived in sacrifices, oblations and pieces of religion. Mundaka subsequently argues that it's dumb and weak, because it makes no difference to the present and post-life existence of man, because it's like blind men leading the blind, it's a hallmark of self-denial and empty intelligence, naive ignorance like children's, a pointless artificial activity. The argument of Maitri Upanishad that all sacrifices in Maitrayana-Brahmane are performed in the hope of finally preparing a man for meditation and bringing him to the awareness of Brahman. So, let this man meditate on the Self after he has placed these flames, and become total and complete.

Maitri Upanishad

In the oldest Upanishads the opposition to the practice is not explicit. At times, the Upanishads expand the task of the Aranyaka with a ritual allegorical and philosophical significance. The Brihadaranyaka, for instance, interprets horse sacrifice practice or allegorical Ashvamedha. It states that by sacrificing a horse, the over-lordship of the world can be acquired. Then it is said that only through the renunciation of the universe conceived as a horse can spiritual autonomy be achieved.

Similarly, the Vedic gods like Agni, Aditya, Indra, Rudra, Visnu, Brahma and others are in the Upanishads equalled with the ultimate, eternal and infinite Braham-Atman, God is identical with the self and is proclaimed to be everywhere in every human being and in every living creature. Ekam Eva Vitiyam or "one and the other and without a second" in Upanishads is the one reality or Ekam Sat of the Vedas. In the Upanishad, Brahman-Atman and self-realization develop as the road to the moksha (free life and freedom).

The thinkers of Upanishadic texts can, according to Jayatilleke, be divided into two classes. One community, which included early Upanishads and some mid- to late Upanishads, was made up of metaphysicians who used rational arguments to empirical experience to formulate their philosophical assumptions and speculations. The second group consists of many Upanishads, who professed theories based on yoga and personal experience. Yoga theory & practice is "not completely absent in the Early Upanishads," adds Jayatilleke. In these Upanishadic theories theory evolved within contrast with Buddhism, as a soul (Atman) is assumed to be the Upanishadic inquiry, while a Buddhist believes that there is no soul, states Jayatilleke.

Brahman and Atman

In the Upanishads Brahman and Atman are two ideals of prime importance. The Brahman is the ultimate reality and the Atman is the spirit. Brahman is the material explanation for what happens, accurate, formal and final. It is the all-encompassing, sexless, eternal, eternal truth and happiness, but the root of all transformation. Brahman, "is the eternal, manifested and non-manifest root, substance, center and destiny of all creation, the shapeless infinite substratum, from which the universe formed." "The creative concept that is known all over the World is Brahman in Hinduism," Paul Deussen says.".

The word Atman means a person's inner self, the souls, the divine spirits and every living thing, including animals and trees. In all Upanishads, the main idea is the Tetman, and its thematic focus is "Know your life." These texts say that not the body, the mind, or the ego, but Atman– "soul," or "self"– is the inner core of every person. Atman is the spiritual essence of every person, its very essence. She's young, old. Athman is what you are at the lowest level of your life.

Atman is the main topic of the Upanishads, but two different themes are expressed. The two are rather divergent. Younger Upanishads state Brahman (the Highest Truth, Universal Concept, Being-Consciousness-Bliss) is the same as Atman, while former Brahman state Upanishads, Atman, but not the same. These somewhat conflicting ideas had been synthesized and merged by Brahmasutra from Badarayana (100 BCE). The Brahman sutras render Atman and Brahman both distinct and non-different, according to Nakamura, a view that was later

called bhedabheda. Koller says that Brahman sutras claim that Atman and Brahman are different on some levels, particularly during ignorance, but that Atman and Brahman are identical and non-different on the deepest level and in the state of self realization. This ancient debate has developed into several dual and non-dual Hindu theories.

Reality and Maya

According to Mahadevan, the Upanishads present two different types of the non-dual Brahman- Atman. The one wherein the non-dual Brahman-Atman is the universe's all-inclusive field, and the other where empirical, evolving truth appears (Maya).

The Upanishads describe the world and human experience as an interplay of Purusha (the universal, unchanging concepts of awareness) and Prak litti. The first is a tribune, the latter as a tribune, and Māyā. The Upanishads describe Atman as "true knowledge" (Vidya) and Mayan knowledge as "not true knowledge" (Avidya and Nescience, lack of consciousness, lack of genuine knowledge).

"The term Maya was translated as' illusion' in the Upanishads, but then it does not include natural illusion," explains Hendrick Vroom. Myth' here doesn't mean that the world is not possible and is simply a human imagination construct. "To suggest, according to the Wendy Doniger" that the universe is an illusion (māyā) is not to say that the world is not possible; it is to say instead, that it is not what it seems, that it is something that is constantly being done. It means to be a reality, but a reality that we live through is deceptive in its true nature "Māyā does not just confuse people about what they claim to know; he limits their understanding more fundamentally.

Māyā is described in the Upanishads as the changing reality and he coexists with Brahman, the hidden true truth. Maya is an important idea for Upanishads, because the texts say it's Maya, which darken, confuses and distracts a person, in the human pursuit of happy and freeing self- knowledge.

Together with the Bhagavad Gita and the Brahmasutras, the Upanishads are one of the three principal origins of all Vedanta schools. The Upanishads have based their various interpretations on the variety of philosophical teachings. Vedanta schools strive to answer questions about atman and Brahman's relationship and about Brahman's relationship with the world. The Vedanta Schools are named after their friendship with Brahman:

There is no distinction, Advaita Vedanta says.

The jīvātman is a of Brahman, according to Vishishtadvaita, and is therefore related, but not identical.

All human souls (Jīvātmans) and matter, according to Dvaita, are immortal and separate beings.

Other schools in Vedanta include Dvaitadvaita of Nimbarka, Suddhadvaita of Vallabha and Bhedabheda of Chaitanya. The philosopher Adi Sankara wrote on 11 Upanishads of mukhya.

Advaita Vedanta

Advaita means non-duality literally and is a monistic theory of thought. This addresses Brahman and Atman's non-dual life. Advaita is the most influential sub-school of Hindu philosophy in the Vedanta School. In reflecting on the Upanishad comments, Gaudapada became the first person to reveal the fundamental principle of Advaita philosophy. Shankara (8th century CE), the Advaita ideas of Gaudapada, have been further developed. King declares that Mā Samukya Kārika, Gaudapadas principal work, is infused with Buddhism's philosophical terminology. King also notes that Shankara's writings are distinctly different from the Brahmasutra, and many of Shankara's ideas contradict those of the Upanishads. Radhakrishnan, on the other hand, indicates that Shankara's view about Advaita was straightforward production by the Upanishads and Brahmasutra.

In the discussions of the philosophy of the Advaita Vedanta, Shankara referred to the early Upanishads to explain the major difference between Hinduism and Buddhism, arguing that the Hindu is Atman (Soul, Self).

The Upanishads contain four sentences, Mahāvākyas, which Shankara used to describe Atman's and Brahman's identity as scriptural truth:

"Prajñānam brahma" – Aitareya Upanishad - "Consciousness is Brahman" "Aham brahmāsmi" – Brihadaranyaka Upanishad - "I am Brahman"

"Tat tvam asi" – Chandogya Upanishad - "That Thou art"

"Ayamātmā brahma" – Mandukya Upanishad - "This Atman is Brahman"

While the Upanishads are supported by many different philosophical views, commentators have usually followed Adi Shankara in seeing idealist monism as the dominant force.

Vishishtadvaita

Vedanta is the second school to be established by Sri Ramanuja (CE 1017–1137) by Vishishtadvaita. Adi Shankara and Advaita School were disagreed by Sri Ramanuja. Visistadvaita is a philosophy of synthesis that bridges the monistic Vedanta Advaita and theistic Dvaita systems. Sri Ramanuja also quotes the Upanishads and says the base of the Upanishads is Vishishtadvaita.

The study of the Upanishad by Sri Ramanuja's Vishishtadvaita is a trained monism. Sri Ramanuja interprets Upanishadic literature in order to teach theory of body mind, "notes Jeaneane Fowler– professor of philosophy and religious studies, who has Brahman as his soul, his inner power, his immortality. The Upanishads are the same qualities as the Brahman according to the Vishishtadvaita School but are distinct in quantity.

The Upanishads are interpreted at Vishishtadvaita School in order to teach an Ishwar (vishnu), who is the seat of all good qualities, with all the empirically conceived universe, as the body of God that resides in all life. The school encourages a commitment to godliness and a daily recollecting of personal god's beauty and love. It brings you eventually to the essence of Brahman abstract. Through Sri Ramanuja's interpretation, "The Brahman in Upanishads is a living reality," Fowler says, "the atman of all life and beings.".

## Dvaita

Madhvacharya (1199–1278 CE) founded the third school in Vedanta, the Dvaita school. The presentation of Upanishads was considered to be profoundly theistic philosophic. Compared to Adi Shankara's arguments for Advaita and Sri Ramanuja for Vishishtadvaita, Madhvacharya says his theistic Dvaita Vedanta is based on Upanishads.

Fowler states: "The Upanishads who speak of the soul like Brahman speak of resemblance and not individuality," according to the school of Dvaita. Madhvacharya interprets Upanishadic lessons of oneself as "entering Brahman," just like a drop in the ocean. It implies duality and dependency for the Dvaita school, in which Brahman and Atman are different realities. Brahman is a separate, autonomous, supreme Upanishad reality. According to Madhvacharya, atman only resembles the Brahman in a minimal, less dependent way.

Sri Ramanuja Vishishtadvaita and Shankara's Advaita school are both non-dual schools of Vedanta; both are premised on the belief that all souls will be able to hope and reach a state of happy liberation.

# Chapter Five

# The Conscious Mind.

The sleeping state is one in which all fourteen organs remain calm and when the self or the soul is not sensitive to sound, touch and other things because of lack of real understanding. And one who knows how to build and dissolve these three states– wake up to dream and sleep– but is itself beyond creation and dissolution is known as turiya– the fourth state of consciousness, turiya.

Awareness is nothing in itself. One is always aware of something; then "about" is important. Knowledge is always objective: you are conscious of something. If nothing is before you, knowledge will collapse– you won't be aware. This state is the sushupti. It is the third state; the oriental religious understanding says it. If no person is identified, the wise man is lost. If there is therefore no external person to be aware of and if there is no mental entity, dream object, if all things break– internal, all dream things are– then drops the awareness? Then you don't know; you're unconscious. Sushupti is the third stage of this unconsciousness.

But it's incredible: it means we're not really conscious, we're just critically aware of it. We didn't know ourselves; we knew only things and artifacts. Our awareness is directed to others; it's not self-centred. Only when another thing is present, I can be conscious. I'm going to go to sleep if nothing is there. Without the target, I have known no subjective knowledge. This is why consciousness is equal to unconsciousness in the third state– it is rendered unconscious. If you don't have a problem, you are ignorant.

This consciousness is therefore a war, a challenge just, a persistent stimulus response; it is no thing in itself. This consciousness is nothing but a struggle. You are not the master; you are not really conscious: you are only constantly forced to be aware. All causes you to realize; otherwise it will be the random act to go to sleep– you will only slip into a coma. Can we call this experience, therefore? It doesn't happen. This state is not self-awareness, it is only a constant tension between you and the world and between you and your feelings. If there's no artifacts and you don't remember... And be unconscious, be unconscious. That's sushupti, the third condition. You can not find it conscious until you overcome it.

The man had no spirit, Gurdjieff used to say. He used to say you have no self, because yourself means self-awareness; otherwise, how can you say you have a self? How could you be a self if

you're not aware? How could you be an individual? So, the teaching of Gurdjieff does not think every man has a spirit. He says, "That individual has the potential to grow and not to grow."

If you are self-aware, you create the person; you become the individual. You're only an entity among other objects if you're not aware of yourself, and nothing more happens there. This is the key point of Gurdjieff's teaching. He says, "There is no entity to recall. Try to remember yourself without anything, without anything else. It's very hard; in some sense it seemed difficult. Recall yourself explicitly, clearly." Without in any way considering anything else, can you recall yourself? Can you remind yourself of that? Can you sound like you?

Wherever you feel, you know about: a son of someone, a daughter, a husband of someone, wealthy or poor, country-owned, safe or sick, but that's all about something else. You know that you are safe. Without a relationship, do you know yourself? Unconnected? Without a background? You only? It is unlikely. We didn't really know each other, we just met in relationship. And this is the miracle: in relation to someone who knows themselves in relation to you, you know yourself. See its nonsense! Someone knows himself for others– and because of him others know themselves.

All are ignorant, but you become wise when you are connected to other ignorant people. You know yourself because you know your name, your address, your place, your country– and you don't know who you are for one moment. This sushupti must be broken up and penetrated into this third state of being unconscious. You must become aware of yourself without any other relation– self-knowledge. The fourth is called the turiya.

We have to distinguish the being from the states. Any state, whether awake, dreaming or sleepless, can not be interchangeable, for the being is what these states are all about. The being is one who passes through all three countries. He can't be identified with anyone; he can't move otherwise. You can't be wake when you associate with dreaming: you can't be wake if you dream, though. You can't go to sleep when you're awake. You pass, but, as you go into and from your home, you go in and out. So, the inside of your home or outside of your house can not be identified. You're moving: you can come inside; you can go out. You pass from sleep to dream, from dream to wakefulness; you move from sleep to dream.

Therefore, this mover should be something else– it's the fourth, and so it's called the fourth. So, no names called... It's never able to shift from the fourth. It could never move from the fourth. When I say this, you have to ask a question: "Am I to sleep this fourth, to dream and other states." This can be grasped very subtly. No, the fourth never goes out, these states come and go– the fourth is always there. Dreaming occurs when winds come across the sky. Mm? The sun rises, then clouds, and the clouds go down. The fourth center in you is the unmoving centre. The dreams come, then objects will be seen, the thoughts will come; then objects will fall, and thoughts will fall, and the fourth one will be in the middle of a deep night. The fourth one will never pass. That is why it was not named; no name is required– the name remains unnamed. The fourth must be penetrated.?

This is not a state, it must be called the fourth state when we speak, but it is not a state. Just three are states; the fourth is beyond them. The fourth one is the being– the fourth one is one's own heart. If you do not hit this 4th nucleus, if you do not know it unless you are focused in it, there is no liberation and there is no happiness. If you are not. Really, nothing is but dreaming. There are plenty of visions, plenty of kinds of visions, but nothing else.

This fourth.... How to get to the fourth? What is this fourth to be achieved? Why is this deep sleep penetrated? Why can this darkness be destroyed? What to do? What to do? The one important thing is first of all to be alert: be conscious of it while you are awake. Be alert of what you do. Walking on the street, then you realize you pass. You should double your consciousness: one arrow conscious of the act of walking, one arrow deep within and conscious of the walker. Listen to me, be aware, double-arrowed: one arrow of your consciousness goes out and listens carefully, the other goes into the hearer.

Mahavira's got a very lovely word. He used a very original meaning as a "listener," a shravak, and gave it a very new shape, a new complexity. He says nothing else is needed if you can simply be the right listener. If you can listen right — samyak shravak. That'll do it a lot. If you can listen carefully with a double focus, then you are awakened, this is enough. It needs no other discipline.

The Buddha used the word, "caution"— samyak smriti, careful treatment. He says anything you do, do it attentively; do it not in sleep, do it attentively, whatever you do. Be awake of it then, in the first state of awaken, consciousness starts to crystallize. You will enter the second state, dreaming, when you have been awake, when you wake up. Then it's not hard. And you can then become conscious of your dreams, so illusions vanish when you become mindful of your illusions. You are conscious of your incredible sleep and the arrow goes on the moment dreams fade. Now be aware that you're dreaming, and you're going through the button, and you're instantly in the fourth. Religion can't be a religion. Religion can not be tradition. It can not be tradition. Religion can not be a religion embraced. Religion is inherently individual: one must always discover it. You have to find it for yourself. There is no intelligence until you ask.

Any information gathered from other people is actually fabricated, false, disappointing. You have to face the facts yourself. You know if you do, that's just like sex. If you haven't loved, you might know all about love, but love isn't understood, because love isn't a real knowledge, an experience. Not even practice, maybe, but knowledge. Experience means everything you witnessed and it's dead now. Experience means something that's over and over with a complete stop. Experience means an ongoing process. You will continue to discover, explore –and it's never over.

Religion is like love:

There's a start, but there's no finish. You must start but never hit it– you hit it. You continue to reach it. You continue to reach, but never before. You can't say, "I've arrived" and you can't stop there. No, never. This is why we call the ultimate quest the holy hunt. We mean by "final" the start, the finish, the end. Instead, it comes to a time when you're lost, but the end hasn't come. However, the explosion is this seeker who is lost.

Not believe, though, unless you ask. Never feel comfortable with words, beliefs, scriptures, unless you learn. If you don't know, keep in mind that you must look and find out, that you must make a journey far away. And that is why faith is the only adventure; everything else is childish. What can be found is only infantile; what can be found is not really the adventure; it does not need bravery to have anything. Only the unlikely requires bravery, only the incontrovertible. You're in an adventure if you search for it. But when you're up for the impossible, it's impossible. The miracle happens as soon as you are ready to take the leap. You're not in a way, you're lost in the hop. And yet you are– you find yourself– for the first time.

State is lost, identification is lost, name and type are lost. The only source left is this rishi: these are the states; these three are the nations. These are the three states. The fourth of these countries is the friendship. These three states come out of the fourth, the fourth is dissolved again and the fourth never emerges from anything and in no other form is dissolved. The fourth is the definition of death, everlasting life, eternal existence.

# Chapter Six
# Meditation

One is to evaluate and break something into its pieces, but not the whole part. They make up the whole, but they are not the same. Without the parts, the whole can not be created. However, the entire is still more, something more than all the components together. The mystery is that plus.

There is a separation of study and research is the knowledge obtained. The same is the confidence. Confidence. This is not a division, but the synthesis that confidence believes. Religion continues to add, complete. And when all is done- nothing is outside, all is included; and all of this, taken as a whole- the divine emerges. So, science can never say there's a god— that's unlikely. Therefore, none should expect that science will conclude that every day there is a god, because the scientific analysis itself can not lead to a complete process. The cycle itself leads to the smallest part- never to the entire part- because it depends on division.

In the universe, science can never become any divinity, because divinity is a kind of perfume coming out of the entire world. It's not math; it's organic. He's not electric, he's real. You can cut me into parts, then bring all these pieces back, but I won't be there. But I'm not a mechanical device, I'm not just collected pieces and put. You put everything again in order. More than all of the pieces there is— something is lacking.

Life by empirical analysis can never be understood. Just material, not spiritual, can be understood by psychology. These are the two knowledge dimensions. If, however, anyone discovers that nothing but matter exists, it implies only that the empirical tool has been used– nothing else. When anyone claims there is nothing, but consciousness alone, it only demonstrates that he uses the synthesis approach– not psychology. Freud was using analysis as a technique, so he could not imagine any spirit or spiritual dimension in man. But now another psychologist, Assagioli, uses synthesis as a tool.: There is no flesh, there is only the soul, there is only consciousness. Whenever someone states matter or consciousness, it indicates that a specific search technique has been employed. Logic is research— love is summary. Logic is analysis.

Then religion was always illogical, and science was always charming. The creation of the ego is to be associated with what you are not. Ego means comparing yourself with something that you aren't. No matter what, no mark is needed. You don't have to be identified with it: it is you.

So, whenever an identification is there, it means that you're not- with something else. You can identify the body, the mind. But as soon as you are remembered, you forget yourself. That's the concept of ego. So is ego forming and crystallizing. Whenever you say "I" you have a name or form, a body or a history, with mind, emotions, memories. There's a certain name. You can say' I' only then. When you are unable to communicate with anything and remain with yourself, you can not say' I';' I' drops only. "I" refers to Identify Name is a pillar of every slavery: you are associated and in jail. Your prison is going to be your name. Be anonymous, remain totally yourself, and then independence remains. That, then, is what servitude is: ego is slavery, ego is liberty. And this ego is nothing but something that you are not associated with. Everyone has his name, for example. Everyone has a nameless birth. Then the name is so significant that you can die for the sake of your name.

What is a name? But it is very important as soon as you are marked. And without name– unknown– everyone is born. Or, everybody is recognized as his own type. You take shape. You stand in front of your mirror every day. What do you see? What do you see? – Yourself? – You yourself? No. No. No. No mirror may represent YOU, only the form with which you are identified. But the insanity of the human mind is such that the shape constantly shifts every day, but never are you disappointed. What was your form when you were a child? What was your shape when you were in the womb of your mother? What was your type when you were in the seed of your parents? Can you recognize the egg in your mother's womb-if a photo has been taken for you? Will you remember so tell, "I'm this?" Would you? Yes, but with this egg somewhere back you must have been found. You've been born– and if you can hear the first yell, can you see it and tell, "This is MY scream?" Yes, but it WAS yours and you have to remember that.

If a dying man will create a song. A constantly changing form-a consistency, but always a transition.... The body changes completely every seven years and nothing, not a single cell, stays the same. However, we still believe: "this is my shape, this is me." And there is no form of consciousness. The form is just something outside, evolving and changing– just like clothes.

This identification is ego. If you are not identified with anything – with name or with form or Where's the ego, therefore–

something? You're next, and you're still not. You are then in absolute pureness but you have no ego. There is nothing, he called it ANATTA. Therefore, Buddha called the ego, not-ego; he named it ANATTA, ANATMA. You can not call yourself "I," you can't call yourself "I," you can't call yourself "I." It really is not possible to use this word AVIDYA. It doesn't mean ignorance; it really doesn't mean ignorance... Because it's only bad ignorance. You know nothing, you're stupid. You know nothing. But this avidya is not a negative thing, it is very clear. It's not that you don't know something, but that you know something that isn't. Alternatively, this avidya is a good idea of something that is not. The "I" isn't– the ego is the world's most non-existence.

It looks very tiny and is totally empty. Avidya means this ego, the given image of yourself, the projective core in you. Avidya is an intrinsic force. It's not just ignorance; it's not something that you don't know; you can construct something that you don't know about. Something that is not can be imagined, something that is not predicted. If the subconscious creates anything that isn't, it's selfish. If these subconscious kills all predictions, all awareness and remains without any projective intervention, then this method is called vidya to remove all predictions. Vidya is not knowledge; yet again, vidya is an aid in destroying everything that produces avidya. It is difficult to traduce Vidya. Vidya is a powerful force in you that can kill the creation of the ego. They are both powerful: avidya produces what is not and vidya removes what is not. So vidya is yoga, vidya is religious science.

So, what does this mean for us as Yoga, Ayurvedics or Meditation??

It is not simply an affair or concern of the dreaming person that our sadhanas for Yoga or spiritual path are to be seen first. It belongs to our inner being, which existed before the birth of this body.

This understanding of the four states and of the self-witness behind them suggests that we are a sight, too. We've had as it were two sight states. The first is the dream state which is a subjective and personal vision of one's own minds. The second is the dreaming state that we share with many other individuals is a common and rational dream.

And our entire life is more than just a form of sleep. There is a lot that we do not know because we know some things in life. Above all we do not know the nature of our own existence or the true meaning of our own presence. We have only a shallow and minimal knowledge, which is bound by duality, error and ignorance. The deep sleep shades the silence, ignorance and indifference and connects the waking and the dream states. Our awakened consciousness is clouded in the night, unsure who we are, why we were born, when we were born and what happens to us after death?

They are generally fascinated with the human body, with the wake state and with the waving ego and are never looking behind them. Naturally, biological, psychological and social needs foster a strong emphasis on this waking state. Even if we have a higher consciousness, it is mainly in terms of the drives of the wakeful mind.

To meditators, this knowledge of the four consciousness states is primarily considered by us to enhance our meditation in waking conditions not only, but also through dream and deep sleep. It is not only the concern of the waking state and the waking ego which should be encouraged, it is also the concerns of the self of the four states, especially our eternal soul which is born in many bodies and in various worlds.

Meditation should be an awakening from the universal dream into the actual and everlasting truth of the Divine Wake, the day of clear light of consciousness. Meditation should be an examination of waking, dreaming, deep sleep, and after, and continues for once, 24 hours a day.

Doing our meditation as the last sleep practice is an effective way of turning dream and deep sleep into meditation. Thus, meditative sleep has been referred to as Yoga nidra or Yogic sleep in which, as a means of absolute transcendence, we consciously join the state of sleep. While deep meditation is much like a deep sleep during the waking state, suppressing the consciousness of the mind and body. We must consider sleep at night as the chance for deep meditation above all the world's illusions.

In total, note that your daily movement from dream to dream to deep sleep and back is a Spiritual journey into consciousness, which you can unlock the secrets of your cosmic consciousness. Every day is a beautiful chance to learn yourself. You only live at a time of one day. But every day is paradise, every day is all happiness and every day is full of gladness.

How to encourage people during meditation?

First, you need to make everyone clear that the patient is ill for a physician; otherwise you need not go to the physician. Therefore, you have to make people realize that they are disappointed, maybe for such a long time, that they forget that they are sorry. If they laughed from their very hearts, they can't remember. They have become machines– they do stuff because it is important to do it, but there is no joy. We live an adventitious life. We are accidental at birth, accidental at marriage, their children are casual and their work is accidental.

Your life does not have any sense of growth and direction. That's why we can't be happy.

And you will first let them know where they are –and almost everyone is in the same situation. Death approaches –you can't even believe that tomorrow you will be here. And your life is a total desert– no oasis has been found, no joy, no joy has been felt– then death will ruin all future possibilities. So, you must first make them aware of their pointless, inadvertent, unhappy lives. You know it, but in many respects, you try to suppress your awareness, because knowing it is a torment continuously. And, to forget it, they go to the cinema. You are going to parties, picnics, alcoholic drinks. All you do, just not to remember the truth of your life, your hollowness and your futility.

That's the key thing– to remind you. Once a person understands all of this, it is very easy to lead him to meditation, since meditation is the only response to all of the people's questions. It may be anger, grief, sorrow, meaninglessness, anguish: there may be a lot of problems, but the solution is one.

Meditation is the answer.

And the best meditation form is just a way to bear witness. There are a hundred and twelve methods of meditation, but observing is an essential part of all a hundred and twelve methods. In my opinion, witnessing is the only way. These twelve hundred are separate witness applications. The main, the spirit of meditation, is how to witness.

You are seeing a tree: There's the herb, you're here, but you can't find one more thing? –You see the forest; you see a witness in you who see you see the herb. It is not just the object and subject that divides the entire world. There's something in both, and beyond that there's meditation. And, in all acts... And I don't want people to sit throughout the morning or in the night for an hour or a half. This kind of meditation will not help, because if you meditate for an hour, you will do the opposite for 23 hours.

Meditation can succeed: it is such a practice to be observed that it can extend over 24 hours of the day.

Don't mark yourself with the eater, feed. There's food, there's the eater so you look here. Move, let your body go, but just wait. Little by little, it's the trick. It's a treat and you can look at small things once....

Crossing this crow... You're listening. You're listening. These two are objects and subjects. But you can't see a testimonial who sees both? – The crow, listener, and there's still somebody who looks at the two. It's a phenomenon so plain. Then you can watch your feelings; you can see your feelings, your moods. You can control your thoughts. You don't have to say, "I'm so sorrowful." Basically, you're a witness, a cloud of sorrow passes over you. You could be a witness. There's rage. You're not always mad– there's no way you can be angry– you're always a testimony. You're never mad. You're just a mirror and the anger come and goes. Things happen, are mirrored, shift-and the reflection keeps the mirror clear, unscratched and clean.

Witnessing is finding your inside mirror.

And once you've found this, wonders begin to take place. Thoughts vanish as you actually observe the thoughts. So unexpectedly you never knew a profound silence. As you look at moods– rage, sorrow, joy– they immediately go away and there is even greater silence. And then the revolt, when nothing is to be done. Then the force of the witness turns against himself, as nothing can stop it; there is no remaining property. It is a beautiful word for "object." It just means what stops you and your objects. It just returns to yourself– to the source when your witness has no object. And this is where you are illuminated.

Meditation is just a journey: the end is always the Buddhahood, illumination. And learning this time is learning everything. Then there's no pain, no anger, no insignificance; life's no tragedy. It is an essential part of this universal whole. And there exists an immense joy for your whole life. The greatest need for man is space. You feel satisfied if someone wants you. But if the whole life needs you, your happiness is limitless. And even a tiny blade of grass requires this life as much as the largest star. Inequality is not a matter of fact. No one can replace you. If you don't exist, life will always remain something less– it will never be complete. The feeling, that you are needed throughout this enormous existence, takes away all miseries. You came home for the first time.

# Chapter Seven
# Understanding the Mind.

The associates are called the panchvarga, or the five classes, the grouping of mind, vital air, desire, nature and virtue. Either knowledge or perception, a living being connected with the panchvarga's roots cannot be free of them. The disease emerging from subtle elements such as the mind and its rest seems to cover the self, and it is referred to as the body seed; it's also referred to as the node or heart complex. and within the consciousness the kshetragya or the field knower is called.

Now the Rishi speaks about mental complexity, consciousness complexity. Why are we a complicated matter? Why is it that there is no innocence or simplicity? Why is all just a knot, a mess, a madness inside? If we can open up a mind, we can only see chaos, anarchy. We handle ourselves somehow, but nothing can be called a universe inside. There's chaos inside, there's just chaos. It seems unlikely, this is a blessing we can handle ourselves. What is the construction of these complexes? How did they come into being? How can we assist in shaping them? And how many are the complexes??

All the complexes are divided into five. The first is the mind. Mysticism in the East has always treated the disease as fundamental illness. It's the reverse of the west approach to life. The Greek brain, which produced every Western thought, always treated the brain as the supreme. Mind is the foundation of Greek thought according to.

Mind is the highest, the mind is the most advanced power for Aristotle. But the culture of the East was an epidemic. That is why science could not be established in the East, for if the mind is diseased, then science can not really be established. The Greek mind could give a boost to Western mental development so that a complex science and scientific knowledge system could be developed. The system is now in place, but the mind is missing, the human being itself. It was very expensive. Machines have evolved, but the maker himself remains hollow and meaningless. Technology has evolved and with this technology we can create a very distinct world– but there is no more interest in creating a different world.

Sartre or Camus as well as others – they anything believe there is no meaning whatsoever in life, there is no sense. Sartre says we are doomed to life; it's not necessary, it doesn't have a purpose, it's all meaningless. Nothing will come from all this effort. Camus therefore argues that the only metaphysical question is suicide. Suicide seems to be the only way for us to be safe and active; all else is meaningless.

This is because, at the end of the day, madness and suicide will occur. At the end, only meaninglessness and a desire to forget it can be in your mind. Therefore, the entire West is now trying to forget about itself-by means of drugs, Drugs and so many more. Life is so pointless that it is in agony to be alive. To know it, that it is too much, that it causes pain— the misery around, the suffering around it and the meaninglessness. So, we should somehow forget about it, and fall into a dream world.

It can support chemicals. You're leaving the world and you've been told to "turn on." Where do you transform on? You really turn to a dream world; it makes sense, you can find a purpose there. You can find beauty and poetry there again, but not consciously if you're awake. And these suggest that these chemicals aid consciousness grow. It's nonsense. These don't allow consciousness growth; they just help the process of dreaming. They just help you to dream more beautifully, to dream more profoundly. They don't help awareness; they help unconsciousness. They help deep sleep and dreaming cycles of SUSHUPTI.

This was because you can't go past this stage with the mind. There's no meaning with your mind; there can't be. Logic exists with the mind, but no meaning; reason exists with the mind, but no existence. With your mind you can create the dead and mechanical, but you lose track of personality, life, consciousness and all other things. Mind, says that rishi, is the first disease in one sense, the fundamental disease. Why is mental illness? – Consciousness is a disease only. Mind is only a knowledge disturbance. It's not your personality, it's only an uprising. There's no stress, no mind at the moment. This is the state of mindlessness– the extension of consciousness. You collapse into yourself: you don't dream; you don't go into predictions. You deliberately come to the core with complete alertness when the consciousness is not there.

Meditation means that you can't be a mind. How can I not be an observer! Meditation means how the state of non-mentality is created. It's not about unconsciousness. Conscious and relentless, without any disruption of the consciousness; conscious without ripples, waves, without vibrations. Conscious as a dark, smooth, quiet pad without ripples, without vibrations on the surface.

Another appears to be disturbed, and then this whole disruption cycle becomes self- perpetuating. Ten more are created by a disturbance and hundred others by these ten. You are in a vicious circle and then self-perpetuated. Something can be achieved with that thought. In other words, you will fly outside and go into the world more. But the farther you go into the universe, the farther you go. The further you go, the more missed the road back. Then you just know there's a room, but there's no way around. And we know that there's always a house; somewhere there's a homesickness. There's a house and you must return.

But there is no way, and we are always trying to find the home with the mind itself. Then we go to the bible, then we go to words, and then we go to philosophy. And then we get lost even further in it, and the track is not found at all. The track can only be identified if you begin to understand and believe that mind is sickness, so that you can't go back with mind; mental can not be used as a means of transportation. It is not a road to consciousness. It is a gateway to the cosmos, to facts– not to subjectivity. So, it's called a disease, it's said to be a complex disease.

The second is PRANA, life itself; instead of it, the desire for life. There's a profound fear– fear of death– and a strong desire to live anyway. The target seems to be life itself.

When life itself is the end, then on the periphery, one must live. Life can not be the end in itself. Something must be more important than life itself; otherwise life can have no meaning. There must be something better than life itself. When you say life is the end itself, life is expected to be pointless, because meaning comes from the outside– from the outside always.

There is something for which you exist– that is why we construct many so-called meanings within us.

Money is given because you live for it, power becomes its importance, reputation becomes its value. You construct definitions, but these are just flawed meanings– because you are really prepared to lose control, money, all if life is in danger. You potentially fool yourself, but the disappointment can never come true. Death is above it; it's not beyond it, it can't be. There are so many feelings of discontent and meaninglessness in the West, therefore. This is a simple corollary of the end of life.

Life comes from something and then dissolves into something else. Life is coming up, then going down and then dissolving. The source of life must therefore go beyond creation. It comes out and goes back as a wave rises and falls into the sea; the ocean is outside the wave. The wave is coming and going; that's the moment, and the next moment goes gone. The stream goes back and forth.

Death is a wave. Life is just a wave. Life is beyond death. Death. Those who are too deeply interested and attached and too passionate about death lose their spiritual source of life.

Meaning is just the outskirts: nature is the heart. This meaning we have called GOD. We called this MOKSHA meaning. We called it NIRVANA life.

This can be grasped rather sensibly. We never really said God exists. They say, "GOD IS EXISTENCE." Those who say GOD does not know what they say. There is man; in like manner there is no God. There are trees, there is earth, there is light, but Allah is not. A tree could go out of existence, man could not exist, the sun could not exist, but God would not exist. God is life; God is IS-

NESS. God. And say that Lord is, therefore, is to contradict yourself.

God MEANS is; God means IS-NESS. This is-nes is life-beyond. Life on the ocean of isthmus is just a wave. So, as water, but not as ocean, we are different. On the outskirts, but not in the middle, we are different. We're one in the middle. So many ocean waves, but they are one in the ocean.

But no wave will conceive of it, because it looks so crazy. What do a wave think of all the surrounding waves as one? – Because one is just dying and dropping when another wave is just rising up. If the waves are one, they will fall at one time and rise at the same time. That's why we are the same. So how are one rich and how is one poor if we are all the same? So how young is one and how old is one? And how does one come into being and how does one die? – Obviously, we have to be different. So how is one smart and not one? And you're beautiful and you're not? – we've got to be other, we got to be different. We don't, though. There are small and large waves, waves that go higher and waves that can not go higher. There are tiny waves. But they are always the same– they are the same in the ocean.

You can not go inside if you are mindful of only your wavelike life; it will then become a disease. And if you know that you are a wave, then you must be afraid, because each wave will die, you are expected to be afraid of death. You can see every wave is dying– up and down, so you're afraid. You don't know your own oceanic nature, you only know the wave nature that means life, that means PRANA.

Thus, the rishi says the second bond, and the second difficulty is the desire for life, the second division of diseases. What does that mean? What does that mean? This means that, if you are to live fully, you must be ready to die. This willingness to die is the basic characteristic of a religious mind. This is the very essence of religiousness: this ability to die. This does not mean a propensity to suicide. This is not suicidal because everyone who commits suicide is suicidal because of a desire to live. This may seem paradoxical– but a Buddha never committed suicide! But Why??

A person who doesn't desire to live, who wants to live, why doesn't he commit suicide? "I'm so indifferent to life, I can't be so happy with death, Buddha would claim. How can I get so excited about death? Both mean the same for me. When life is– all right. A buddha all right. If death is– all right. He can't pick. Whenever someone commits suicide, they actually enforce living conditions. He says that life should be like that; I commit suicide otherwise." This woman I must get, I have to get that letter, I have to get it and that. I will live only under my conditions if I don't get there. So, if my expectations are not met, I will die. "This desire to die still isn't ready to die. He's still frustrated. It takes so much energy and life, it's so full of desire that even criteria are placed. This death is only a revenge, only a revenge against life, because life can not satisfy its demands:" I will destroy life if life is not what I want it to be! "It's vengeance, it's violence.

So, if I say that I am ready for death, it doesn't mean a hunger for life, and you still feel welcome, receptive. Anything that occurs is ready –even death. The disease is caring for life. This readiness to die unites the hunger for life. The third challenge is wishes. We don't exist, we exist in wishes. We don't really exist, we exist in fantasies, in the universe at all. Our life here and now, where our wish is arrowed, is always elsewhere. It could be anywhere, but never here. Never here, because wish takes time –wishes can not be here.

In the present moment, do you want anything? When you want, you want the future; here and now you can not wish. There's no desire here and now, no desire chance. Desire wants space – time is space. Desire wants something else from here– desire can only exist then. The bridge operates as a bridge: the bridge needs two banks; on this branch only a bridge can not exist. How is the bridge possible? It must be the other one; there must be the other branch. This is the only way to achieve the bridge. Desire builds a bridge between here and there.

And when you go there, you will live in an inner strain, an inner agony, as soon as you have lost this time. And you will never be eternal, in wishes, desires, just looking for the other side. And you will never be universal. Even if you can come to the other side, you'll want the other coast again. There can be no shore to complete– desire frustrates itself. The thoughts are we. Can you find something that is not a need in you? It's love, even when you pray; even if you meditate its desire; even when you speak of the spiritual, it's desire. We transform all into desire. This is the condition that we can foresee nothing unwillingly.

Buddha used to maintain, "No God." So, he himself was one of the divine's most existential proofs. He was the divine's perfect argument; his existence was divine. And he had been saying that there was no God. Sariputta asked him one day, "Why do you still maintain that there's no God? –That when you are, we all know that God is. A person like you, who denies God, seems contradictory. It seems contradictory, because your proof, you're sufficient! We need no argument, so why do you deny it??"

The Buddha said, "I deny it that I don't like the notion that God is made a want thing. When I tell God is, you'll start desiring,' Then I have to get, then I have to get there.' Because God is something you can't want because you can't do it by wants." "And he'd add," No, but then there is no existence. "Why? Just because you start desiring it if there's life after death. They'd add," Is paradise here? Can we have joy? "The Buddha is going to say,' No. Just suffering is prevented, there is no joy. He was a special genius who saw the want phenomena, the want tricks and the wisdom of desire. He would say, "No, there's absolutely no happiness; just cease to suffer." Why? – Because when you're told the bliss, you continue to want it.

We turn all into love. We have a conversion and transformation process. Put in everything, and it will become like desire. We may even want unwillingness. I found people coming and asking, "How can I be unwilling?" How reluctant to ask– how reluctant to be– how unwilling to be! But we're trying to convert. It's the illness, it's the disease, really. See the illness, see the truth so inquire not the "how." Look at the fact: it is. Live with the fact. Live with the fact. Answer mindful of the function of your subconscious, and how it all transforms into desires. In this moment of consciousness, desire ceases. And you are here– this very moment when there is no desire. This moment is the doorway to the infinite. The moment is the doorway to the divine– to nirvana.

# Chapter Eight

# Phenomenology, Experiences, and States of Consciousness

What do holons from the inside look like? What you feel right now, whatever happens.

It gets a bit more complicated from there, however. The disparity between systems and states is one of the important differences AQAL highlights. In the most general sense, "Systems" is simply just another word for any degree (in any quadrant). Every level of a line has a patterned structure or. The patterned wholeness or phases are the constructs examined in structuralism and developmentalism, when perceived from without in an objective way. There are therefore, where Loevinger is concerned, certain essential constructs (or levels) of the ego's developmental line: "conformist, cautious," "individualist," etc.

(Such structures or levels occur in sequential phases so we often compare "structures" and "stages," but theoretically they are distinct, so we won't equate them in this discussion. Inelegant as it may be, when we mean the sequence of the development of zone 2 structures in the psyche, we are thinking about structural level. The development stages are Loevinger, Kegan, Selman, Perry, Broughton, etc.)

In this section we want to look into and compare and contrast the states of consciousness with those of consciousness– sterile as it may initially look like, this relationship is perhaps the key to the understanding of the nature of spiritual experiences (and therefore of the role played by faith in the modem and the postmodern world). Let's start with this humble and dumb introduction.

We said Zone 1 in the UL (indoor view of a T) is just what I hear, think, and feel right now. I should explain my present and immediate perceptions and fears in clear first-hand terms, and I would do just that by several forts of phenomenology ("There is a sensation of heaviness, heat, discomfort, lightness, affection, concern, exaltation and momentary experiential flashing etc."). These are all anomalies in Zone I approaches, some of which study other types of inner experience known as exceptional states.

What I experience instantly, as a first person, includes what often are called "phenomenal states" in addition to basic "contents," or "immerging experiences" – such as a feeling, a mind, an instinct, an image, etc. I never experience specifically something like "a conscious machine," although I may be in the stage at which all my thoughts are currently unknown to me within this setting. Structures can not be discovered only by zone 2 techniques, and meditation or contemplation of any kind can not be used to discover them. On the contrary, States are, under different circumstances, directly available for information. I have states, not structures, I realize.

Most of us realize consciousness nations, and so are the great principles of wisdom. For example, Vedanta gives five key natural consciousness conditions: waking, dreaming, deep sleep, testimonials (turiya) and nondual (turiyatita).

Altered or non-normal states, like exogenous states (i.e. induced drug) and endogenous States (i.e. qualified states such as meditative states), also occur in addition to regular or ordinary states.

Increased conditions are often known as peak encounters, both normal and non-ordinary.

There is a mapping of countries like, human, exogenous and endogenous states and possibly, of the great traditions.

Some of the meditation maps are extraordinarily complex, but are focused on Zone-I methods and guidance (e.g. zazen, shamanic travel, central prayers, vipassana) and can be verified by those interested in training as phenomenological experiences.

It is an interesting question (and that will be revisited, as this is one of the main areas of integral post metaphysics) that phenomenological encounters ('see, what seems like limitless light and love') have real ontological parallels ('there is divine foundation of being'). The psychedelic mapping Of Stan Grof is also a zone I mapping for those interested (which's why no zone 2 phases are included in any of its mapping).

Many major cultures have developed a complex psychology that goes along with these systems, and even if the specifics don't hold us back, let me highlight some significant features. The points that I am about to sum up are challenging and hard to prove in themselves. But for the moment we are just going to assume them. I will use Vedanta and Vajrayana as an example. We will have to begin with a complicated terminology (although Neoplatonism would be just as well).

The meditative states are different versions of natural states according to every one of them. For example, meditation with type is a variation in the dream status (Savikalpa Samadhi, for example), and meditation without form is a variation in deep sleep without form (nirvika / pa samadhl). In addition, three primary natural states (waking, dreaming or sleeping) accompanied by specific energy or' body,' (free gross body, subtle body, and causal body are said to sustain the testimony / nondual states) (e.g. Nirmanakaya, Sambhogakaya, and dharmakaya, respectively).

Although the terms "dirty," "subtle," and "causal" literally mean only species or energies (in the UR), we also apply to the corresponding state of consciousness (in the UL). Therefore, 5 major, natural and/or meditative consciousness states can be referred to as: extreme, subtle, causal, testimonial and non-dual states of consciousness. I frequently refer to 3, 4 or 5 separate states of consciousness, as practices do themselves– all 5 of which are intended).

The inference is clearly that for those of you who stopped trying to understand what I said somewhere in the middle of that essay, all men and women have at least five major states of consciousness which can all be encountered explicitly according to the great traditions of wisdom.

Subtle dream states, as I can experience in a vivid dream or a lively visualization exercise or in certain forms of meditation of shape, as in a vivid "day dream," or in the exercises of visualization;

Ever-present non-dual consciousness, which is not so much a condition as ever-present, is a state of deep sleep and of the kinds of shapeless contemplation and perception of total openness or emptiness; witnessing states or "the witness"— which is a witness to all other states, such as a capacity for unbroken concentration in a waking state and a potential for a clear vision.

The Vedanta and the Vajrayana hold that all human beings have access to these states and their corresponding bodies or realms by virtue of' the precious human body.' This means that all humans at almost every stage of growth, also in their babies, have access to these major states, simply because even the babies are waking, dreaming and sleeping.

That's a very, very, very important point, that we will come back to.

(As a sneak preview, since the main contours are always present, you can have a full experience of a higher state but not of a higher stage. For instance, work in the awareness-raising stage of Jane Loevinger continues to show that you literally can not have a peak experience in a higher structure, such as the autonomous, but you can have a peak have of a major, subtle, causal, observing, or nondual state of consciousness. Exactly how we're going to want to return to these two suits together.)

While they are naturally and instinctively accessible to all humans, some of them are extensively educated or studied, and then they hold some surprises.

Trained States: Meditative and Contemplative States

Though all people are said to be available for the greatest states of being and consciousness, this does not mean that they can not be further educated and exercised at every point. State preparation is a particularly advanced zone I technique that is extended to extremely advanced forms in East and West grand meditative practices.

Normal states generally show no development. There are dream states, but none of them go anywhere. Many rates are found in normal structures and the most altered states. We just come and go, as most states do — whether a thunder-like emotional state or a weather state. Therefore, you can not be intoxicated and sober at the same time, most states of consciousness are exclusive. And even in advanced stages, normal states exist– still buddhas are waking, dreaming and sleeping (although they are non-dual).

Nonetheless, some states can be trained and if this means treatment— like many ways of meditation and reflection— then these states appear to be formed in series, and they tend to follow the natural order from gross to subtle to causal to nondual states.

That is why extraordinary conditions in many meditation settings, from major phenomena ("I see rocks," "the rocks"), to subtle phenomena ("I see light and joy, I feel vast love," "there is only great darkness and an endless abyss,") are represented in my direct and first-person experience as nondual to causal phenomena (the divine void and reality are not two. "These are not first person (seen in zone 2), but first-person countries (zone 1). These are first person programs.

If states arise in some kind of sequence, call them phases (compared to phases in structure). Since states are much more amorphous and fluid than structures by their very nature, this stage series is very fluid and fluid— you could also peak higher states (Although they are typically transient, without additional training –altered states or temporary peak experiences –they can be converted into what are known as plateau experiences through further training). So, if you're on a particular stage, it can often happen momentarily, but don't hold it as an experience on the plateau.

Moreover, as research shows time and again, you can not bypass structure stages, nor can you reach a higher level in structures. At the other hand, research shows time and again that structure phases are relatively discrete stages or rungs in development. As for these stages progressively moving from gross experience to subtle experience and causal experience to nondual, you may open virtually any meditation or contemplation manual, East or Western, and you will find a list of meditative or spiritual experiences that basically unfold in this order with very specific references. (We will return soon to the relationship of states and structures.). One immediately thinks of the inner castles of St. Theresa, of St. John Of the Cross ' remarkable maps of the Church of St. Gregory of Nyssa (whose distance from purification), the path of enlightenment and the path of reconciliation is as short and brief a overview as you'll find— cleanse the gross body, by discipline, and yet the gross mind through concentric focus. Their tale is as short and succinct as they are found.

It could be that Daniel Brown (reported in Wilber, Engler, Brown, et. al., Transformations of Consciousness— Traditional and contemplative prospects for creation, 1986; 2006 reissue) has studied some of meditation practices with the greatest care. The root texts and primary remarks are performed in three major meditational practices: The Yoga sutras OF Patanjali, the Visuddhimagga OF Buddhaghosa, and the Mahamudra Nges Don. zerof Bkra shis mother rgyal. In a way, these are both the Hindu and Buddhist pillars.

Brown pointed out that the meditative direction in all of them went through a similar basic cycle of contemplation, both variations on gross preliminary and training and subtle observations Of luminosity and light, then changes in formless absorption or black-near causes, and then a failure to achieve nondual awareness (and then further potential "post illumination" refinements). The thorough care and research, including the reading of the texts in their original languages, has made Brown'.

We called for transformations of conscience co-published by Brown and Engler.

If we were to focus on his own extensive work in the contemplative states in the early Childish fathers, Harvard theologian John Chirban. The work we did. Also, since these are state stages and not structural stages, there may be a great deal of fluidity, transient skippers, high levels of experience in higher state (not structure), and so on. It also showed gross phenomenon to subtle light to causal darkness and nondual union. "But as states are mastered, the general progression was indeed gross to subtle to ungual.

States are difficult to photograph pictorially; we are going to settle for cloud-like regions. Figure 8 illustrates the standard development in meditation over a complete training course Meditative education lasting between 5 and 20 years. What we are seeing is a progression Of Wakefulness via gross to subtle to causal towards nondual— a progression Of Wakefulness from its usual restriction in the waking state, to a Wakefulness that continues into the dream state (at which point, lucid dreaming is prevalent) and/or intermittent meditative states, and then into the causal formless state (by whatever name), at which stage states Of advanced mindfulness practice, including cessation, are possible, and/or a very tacit awareness trying to extend into the deep sleep state, so that a Wakefulness is personally witnessed even in deep dreamless sleep (there is

EEG concrete evidence Of patterns in very sophisticated meditators consistent with this claim). All subjective states were made Object of The Witnessing Presence at that point, at which point Nondual union or even identification with a previous ground is often mentioned. Just what a "divine land" entails... ok, you know exactly what it means, but in the light of fundamental meanings, we will come back and explore this awakening.

We have discussed consciousness systems and states. The 64,000-dollar issue is, how do they relate? They may be the quintessential contributions of the contemplative approaches to UL (zone-I reflection and contemplation) and the traditional approaches to UL (zone-2 structuralism and genealogy) respectively. And this takes us back to our initial question, indeed: Why can you sit for decades on your meditation mat and never see anything like the Spiral Dynamics stages? And why you can study Spiral Dynamics until the cows come home and never get satori?

Zones 1 and 2: Zen and Spiral Dynamics

One of the things which I'm going to seek to do during the entire essay is give a very brief overview of well-known and respected methodologies, and then suggest how they can be successfully integrated in the AQAL approach. We begin with Zen and Spiral Dynamics and the above.

The work Of Clare Graves is based on Spiral Dynamics, one of the great pioneers of Zone 2 science. The model was based on research original with university students who had one question: "Describe the actions of a human organism that is psychologically healthy." Following an old-as-Baldwin traditional zone2 process, Graves found answers to his request, which eventually prompted it to formulation of a development system. Spiral Dynamics, based on Graves ' work, refers both to a' MEME' identified by the specified' systems or values, meme,' and to a' core intelligence.' Graves and SD talk about 8 levels / status of this low adaptive intelligence (all terms are from spiral dynamics directly):

Level 1 "Survival Sense" staying alive;

Level 2 "Kin Spirits" Magical; safety and security;

Level 3 "Power Gods" Impulsive; egocentric; power and action;

Level 4 "Truth Force" Purposeful; absolutistic; stability and purposeful life; Level 5 "Strive Drive" Archivist; multiplicity; success and autonomy; Level 6 "Human Bond" Communitarian; relativistic; harmony and equality; Level 7 Integrative systemic; "Flex Flow"

Level 8 "Global View" Holistic; experiential; synthesis and renewal;

Most people with spiral dynamics have difficulty understanding the fundamental nature the idea that this mechanism is part of a larger AQAL structure, so let me suggest this thought experiment and see if it helps. Let's just say that you're grown, purposeful at level 4. You read the book, you store all 8 or 8 MEMES examples, talk to the teacher and the classroom. You read them. You take the final exam and you are asked to describe and correctly describe the 8 layers of values systems. The exam will give you a perfect 100.

The explanation that levels 5, 6, 7 and 8 can be described– although only level 4 itself– is because they are described outside or zone 2 descriptions. These are depictions of different realities in 1st person. You can get a perfect 100 on the test because you can store TT-. These descriptions of the person, although you do not have the descriptions on the top level. you have put them yourself. And there are plenty of people now dreaming of green turquoise values, etc.

Speaking of another analysis now. That says: "Please explain Level 8 experience in the immediate and first-person language that it feels directly right now," including an oral review in the same manner. You will totally flunk that check if your self-sense is really at level 4. The 3rd person examination can be passed, but the 1st person exam can be flunked.

In other words, if you follow the steps of SD, you can see those steps outside of them (or the third person), but you can't turn them into stages higher than what you are at. That is not a failure of the system. This is precisely what descriptions of zone 2 are—namely descriptions of the third person and conceptual formulations of 1 HP.

Therefore, you will not necessarily be modified by studying Spiral Dynamics for years. It needs Yd-person knowledge and not the self-identity of the first person. Again, this is NOT a flaw of the model, what Zone 2 approaches does EXACTLY (or 3rd party approaches the truth of the first person). I am a big fan of Clare Graves' work and the very open way it is created by Spiral Dynamics by Don Beck and Christopher Cowan. As the best simple introductory interface, I still suggest SD. And of course, don't know how much to make many of the original Graves research accessible to a large audience; Chris Cowan and Natasha Todorovic did a great job.

As for the change itself: How and why people are evolving, shifting and improving are one of human psychology's great mysteries. No one knows the truth. There are many theories, many reasonable assumptions, but little real explanation. Of course, this is an extremely complex subject, which I'm going to finish with this section for the moment.

So, let's presume you decide to take meditation at whichever point of Zone 2 you are. This is an adventure for 1st person, not least YD-person. You begin to have a series of experiences if you take some serious form in reflection or meditation successfully. Because these are meditative interactions and states, the formal stadiums of most zone 2 solutions are not quite rigid. But usually they will produce waves of consciousness that are gross to subtle, causative to nondual, as in tables 2 and 3.

The Ten Ox-Herding pictures are the best known representation of these meditative phases in Zen. These are the phases that demonstrate the overall course of Zen training as well as the moment-to-time progress of any training level. In one sense, it is a stage of careful deployment and training which forces awakening from the traditional confinement to a waking state, and into an awakening of subtle dream phenomena (Savikalpa, god, enlightenment) and causal phenomena (Nirvikalpa, formless darkness at night— this is the ox-herding image of a wide- spreading circle — and then the ever-present nondual B in one sense.

As noted, these are general variations in Daniel P. Brown's zone I states. In its Variety of Meditative Expressions (a book called purposely for William James's great variations of religious experience), Daniel Goleman has given a more general overview of these state-stages, reflecting Goleman's intuitive understanding, I believe, that both of the books are representative of the same area-I technique– phenomenology in the broader sense.

Now to the question of sixty-four thousand dollars: how is the Zen phases related to the Spiral Dynamics??

# Chapter Nine

# Understanding the Body of Man

Sheath set consisting of nourishing food is called the annamaya kosh or the food body in the form of the physical body. The 14 winds, including vital strength, are also known as pranayama kosh, or the vital body, which flow through the dietary body.

Now we must go to the corpses for an examination. Man is not one body; man has a large number of bodies– corporeal layers. The body that we know is the outermost, there is a different body inside, and a different body inside. These layers were split into five by Rishis. The first is called the physical body, the food body. We are usually attached to this body. We are profoundly explained by the actual illusion. You will not be able to move into this connection on the physical body. Why this relation, however? – We don't know there's another; we've never known that there's another one inside this body. This body is so solid, that you can't get a glimpse of it. This power of the body means that we use foods that solidify it. This body can also be made transparent, just as you can see a glass body in it.

The change in diet will improve the physical body's qualities. Nutrition is also a qualitative object and not just energy. Food is not a fuel alone; it adds more than heat– it gives you openness or non-transparency. You can mutate your perception of this phenomenon and have another type of body altogether. This body is not that difficult to change because it is a movement, it changes at all times; it is a mechanism, not a static thing. It's a method. You had another body as soon as you came here; now the body changed. It changes constantly at all times; it's fluvial, shifting, and evolving– it's not static.

Though you change direction, the body jumps; it only has to change direction. You should be conscious that whatever you eat must not make your body heavy. It must be so. This weight is not about weight: you feel weightless sometimes, as if you can float. Therefore, the food that can make you feel weightless is the right food. The food you feel burdened with is not the right food. You can't fly in the earth because of all non-vegetarian food. You have an inner feeling that you can levitate, you can only exit gravity Vegetarian food.

If it is not gravitational, food is right. It's fine if you can sense non-physical. Actually, the body still hurts when it's warm; only then do you sense the body if you feel big. If the body isn't warm, you're physically fat. Therefore, when you're ill, when your body is damaged, you feel anything; you don't feel it when it's safe. If there is no headache, you feel your head only, there is no brain. There is only one way to define wellness in a positive manner: if you do not feel your body, you are safe. The more you worry, the sicker you are, because you don't have to hear it when your body's really safe. There's only pain. And it must be some sort of pain, if you even feel pleasure. Pleasure is never experienced because there is only a perturbation. Never really is quiet heard, just noise. And if you start feeling quiet....

Genuine, genuine silence doesn't hear. Really, it's quiet when you don't hurt any noise. If you don't feel your body, that means you don't feel trouble; you're balanced. Therefore, the sense of physicality is safe. Any food that gives you a sense of physicality is fine, is good food. So be discriminative; be discriminative knowingly. Don't eat anything that reflects you more, make you a body more. Go on to do away with anything that gives you a corporality and then you start to turn your body into transparency. That might seem paradoxical, but it's real. If you're safe you're rejected– illness and unhealth make you want. This is one of the fundamental differences between East and West thinking. In the west, you say you are safe if you are overflowing with desire. But they have a very superficial understanding this desire is a disturbance. Something is incomplete, and the need is also incomplete. There's a need to satisfy something that's incomplete. But you are so full– the process is so complete– that you are so safe that there is no need. But it is so full.

You're incomplete because of ambition. There is something somewhere still missing; there's something still missing; still you sense an ambition.

This means disease or sickness: a vacuum. Health means, there is no more room, so much fulfilled. There is no internal room; so, an individual is really safe and unwanted, and a person who is really safe is uncaring. Both of these are connected: being a body is desirable, being wilful is heavy on the body. As though it wasn't, make the body. The less you are, the better; the more you are, the more down you go. You can only become a pier, and there are many- only pierces. You just feel wake when your body needs something; otherwise you sleep. If the body wants, it feels alive, then it meets the demand– it falls back in sleep again.

One should create an organization that has requirements but not wants. Human needs: anxiety and obsessions are demands. Wants mean that you are addicted; master is the body. All austerity was not intended as suicidal process, it was not masochistic– it truly was an internal move, it truly was a power change.

When a buddha fasts, the body must not be killed; demands must be removed. Understand very well that when a buddha fasts, he does not break his body but changes the strong place, who is the master. You can not go inside the body, otherwise you will not be the master. The master is external. How are you going to go in? You're only a slave, and the master must be around. You have to change the control place; the body has to be a slave. A bondwoman has needs, but no claims; a bondwoman has needs, but no commandments. The control shall remain the master and the master shall be indoors rather than outdoors. The wealthier the king, the more independence you have. So, when a buddha is fast, the seat of power must be changed. The body will be battling– nobody can lose so easily the energy, the lord, the sovereignty– but I'm not going to fulfil your needs, but your demands. And for thousands of years you have been living with the body as the lord. The body was never questioned and so the mastery was normal. It became such an old habit that the body could not even conceive it. Are you master? You're master? You were the slave forever. Ever! You've gone insane? Orders were given by ME already! You've always been watching.

Austerity says, TAPASCHARYA says, TAPAS means you are now unwilling to continue with this status quo. The body will war: the battle is not really inside; the fighting is external. But the body is a very subtle and wonderful mechanism: if you have the will it adapts to anything – the greater the will, the faster you adapt the body. "Mastery now is lost" starts thinking, and the body really gets better when the Mastery is lost, because it's normal now.

The dominance of the body is absolutely unnatural; it is not- even for the body- good because the body is unconscious and demanding; the body doesn't discriminate and goes on demanding. Awareness is made a slave and material needs, mechanical, are the master.

This is the most serious accident; the most profound suffering mankind has had. But in a certain way it had to, because of the animal life we have produced. Via animal life we have evolved. It doesn't take Darwin to explain that- we all knew it. The body needs to be the boss, because an animal has no consciousness. Nobody else claims to be master- the body must be the lord. But when there is consciousness inside, the body continues, mm? – Like an ancient dress. You will change it. You must. You're not in the world of animals now; you're not animals anymore. Austerity means that the state of animalhood has passed now we say. The misery one encounters in austerity is only an agony of birth- nothing else. And this suffering is good and good because transformation is the product of this suffering.

But as a masochist, it must not be done- this is completely different, it's a very ill thing. You can let and enjoy your body. You are suicidal if you like it: it's not austerity. Then it is not austerity, so you're a very weak, aggressive person, really. You can't abuse anyone, so you abuse yourself. You can easily become a masochist, a sufferer. It's not austerity; it's very rare, it is a mental case.

Of the hundred and ninety nine percent of people who undergo austerity are masochists, but they can mislead; they can fool others and they can also deceive themselves. It is pointless to disappoint others but to disappoint one is rather dangerous. You can be deceptive. The argument to be made is that you don't like suffering; you will take it as a necessary measure. You should go through it as a joy, a catharsis, a transition and as a mutation. You must go through it as a purity. It must be remembered, but it must not be enjoined! Which is the thing: if you want it, it's not austerity; it's folly.

That's the point: don't like pain, because it's abnormal. Pain is natural, but it is another thing to accept it as a requirement, as an inevitable. Go through it, embrace it, don't enjoy it. This is what you must do, for one day, you must show your dignity because you have animal heritage. You have to show yourself against the animal heritage. You have to remind your body that it's not the lord, now. And the body is modified once it is learned. And the body is liberated from its intolerable obligations. It CANNOT be the master because it has no consciousness; It is a mechanical device which is automated.

The body is an automatic device and therefore continues to operate. If you make it the master it continues without any comprehension, bigotry, intelligence. It's like a computer with a technical intelligence: it continues... It goes on asking. It goes on asking. It has an integrated challenging process, but without any awareness: without any intelligence, it tells you when you're hungry, what to eat, what to do. But all that is electronic-repeatedly. This system. This is why a person who lives with his / her body thinks life is a boring thing, because his / her body can only repeat it; Therefore, we repeat the same thing every day. It is a circle, a shut circle: the same things, the same requests, the same wants, the same desires– the body repeats and repeats, and in the end, you are only boring but nevertheless nothing can be done. The body demands the same thing, even if you feel bored, once again the second day, and you must supply it because you were never in command.

The first, the main layer– the most visible one, is this physical layer. When you know that you are a slave unnecessarily and don't have to be, then deliberately change your body habits. Move from time to time. Change the power seat; be controlled more. So, give the body everything it wants, but never conquer any addictions. It will be unpleasant at first, but it is a pleasure when you're beyond the body and the master. And it's one of the greatest possible joy when you're on the throne.

Two things aren't matter and money. Matter is only energy; electricity is merely matter-one thing is two states.

The second corpse is the vital one. The vital body is the energy source, the body of power, or anything we want to use– the bioenergy body. It isn't a material thing, it's energy, one thing is certain. Nevertheless, energy can be converted into matter and matter into energy.

Power means that it doesn't change indefinitely. Power means waves, colourful. Living is life.

A tree has two bodies, skeletal and living, rather than just a physical body. Any energy flows, and a tree is sometimes more alive and at times less alive. Also, scientists are now prepared to accept that the tree is more alive when someone is close to an arboreal tree. And the tree is sad and less alive if one is next to the tree that doesn't love it. The whole garden is happy when the gardener comes in. And it's not just a poem; it's a scientific reality now. It's always been a fiction, but not a poem; it's a scientific fact. When a person who loves a tree is next by, the tree is different, and computers can now recognise the difference. It's more alive; it feels better– passion fluctuates. Vice versa, too. Vice versa. When you love trees, you are more, because they are reciprocal. You love trees. You're not just the same when you're next to a plant. If you have love, you have the opening and the bloom and, in a communion, you are deeply linked.

You can cleanse this vital body and it becomes translucent if it is cleansed, and then look beyond. How is she cleansed? PRANAYAMA's cleansed. It is cleaned if a deep breathing system is available. Inside your lungs less carbon dioxide and more oxygen in you-the more energy you make. Simple vibrations can also cleanse the essential body. You make many uncleanness's for your precious body in a crowd. Therefore, when you return from a crowd, you feel a bit less than you do. You get more alive from the crowd, far away from the man to nature, since there are no sinner trees, no sinner's seas, no sinner's heavens.

But the guy has splits, so you're drawn into a crowd! It's depleted your money. You dropped to a lower standard. But there are others– few, very few– that believe that you were packed with; you were full, you were vitalized. To be in business, in communion, in contact with someone who is responsible to your life is what SATSANG is about– this is meant to be similar to a master. No verbal communication is needed; no communication is required externally. Just to be polite and nearby... Just to be free, near, and your vital body grows. It continues to be more beautiful, cleansed.

Look for a company that is clear for your precious body. And even a dead master can help sometimes; even the place can help, the bodhi tree. For 25 years Buddhists have always wanted to save this tree-the same one. Not just entourage; not only superstition; not only a shrine, mm? There are more subtle explanations for saving the one; Buddha was once next to it and the tree took some Buddha. The tree was closely connected with the buddha; the tree itself has a rather subtle Buddhahood. Now, with a specific vibration it vibrates. No other tree vibrates like that on this planet, can not.

It is a rare tree, a rare occasion: for days and nights Buddha walked around. It was Buddha who lied, ate, stood... And Buddha can not afford to be compassionate, and Buddha can not help. The fruit was an ever-growing companion; and the very spirit was imbued by the fruit. And this tree is still completely different today! When you are there and open, you're in the presence of the Buddha himself again, in a subtle way. So that shrines can help, temples can assist, mosques can assist, Samadhis can also help. It's best not to be in your lifetime, even the person lives in the business. If you can feel vitally charged, it's easier to be in company with a dead man.

Remember, then, also remember this: stop everything that destroys your precious body. And a lot is devastating. In a cinema hall, not only is the theatre the film that destroys you, but the whole crowd destroys you more deeply. The film is significant. And it's a special crowd– it's not a crowd, it's a particular crowd– with a common mind with certain steel bodies. You kill more of you. It isn't really a game, the movie can't destroy you much, but the crowd... And they're always in very fast attentive mood for three hours– it's very risky because you're vulnerable. By opening your eyes, you are now open for three hours! Everything can reach you and just bad vibrations are all around you– they go inside. You have a very weakened vital body when you're out of a movie hall, coming out of a temple. Be conscious, however, that the second, essential body is not only mindful of the physical body and its purification.

The third one is called the consciousness, the subconscious. The third is the mind. The sixth is made up of myths. Nevertheless, the experience of yoga believes that thinking is not just feelings, it is things, it's substantial; it is. They have a very vague life of their own, but they exist. And if an idea hits you, you change your mind; you feed it. And we don't know this, that the mind is fed every moment, so we give something, without any choice– it's just a mess.

When the self– residing within the food-body– thinks of things such as sound, smell, touch and so forth, through the instrumentality of the 14 organs, the vital body is known as the manomaya koshu or the intellectual body. If the self, together with these three bodies, understands intelligence, the kosha or the knowing body is called vigyanmaya. When the self dwells in its unconscious and causative ignorance, in union with these four bodies-food, vital body, mental body and knowledgeable body-it's called the anandamaya or blissful bodies.

Everything we keep giving our minds, we just think it should be kept busy; that's all. The mission itself is a target. You shouldn't be unoccupied, so read anything, listen to anything, see anything, go on... Do something with the mind! Do something with the head! We are vulnerable to it, therefore, whatever it is. This is fatal because then you create a confused head-body with inconsistencies and endless inconsistencies. It's very complicated. And this is why there is a great deal of pain, stress and suffering inside. This is why the mind is crazy.

Psychologists now agree that there really are two forms of disorders: one is regular anomalies– another is pathological abnormality. There are therefore two kinds of foolish people: one who are mad and socially accepted– the other is stupid in their individual whims. But everybody seems mad. And it is that our minds-body never thought that an inner harmony, an inner music, is important. Thoughts should not contradict themselves; thoughts have to be harmonious and in a certain inner balance;

otherwise you become just a mob– you are a mob.! C.J. C.J. Jung understood that nobody had a mind: everybody's many people; everybody's polypsychical. We're continuing to talk about "my mind "– never talk again! You are only a multitude, you are not even a group, you are also a multitude, and not a crowd, but a warring crowd.

The guy is like a gate with so many slaves, Gurdjieff used to say but the master is gone out. And it's been out so long that the slaves forget that there's a master right now. Then, when someone goes through the palace... And it's so amazing that everybody wants to ask who it belongs to. Every slave on the door says, "It is mystery. Slave. I'm the owner." But the same person passes another time; someone else is at the door and asks, "Who's this palace? The entire city is puzzled," Who is the master? Who's the master?" "He says, "He's mine." I'm every slave, everyone says, "I'm the Owner." "Such is man's state, Gurdjieff used to say. Every thought that goes through, including on the surface, becomes the master; and the master sleeps or has gone a long way and is not returned. And it was so many years ago...."

We've got no will, therefore. When we're a crowd, we can't have a will. You want to do something, so you assume not to do something the second time. And you're not definitive for the third moment, or even not– you're always indecisive. You assume you will be up at 4 a.m. in the morning; at 4 a.m. you say to yourself, "It's not important!" On the surface of your mind is another girl, not you-that same one who has not decided is here. In the morning, at 8 a.m., you start repenting, "Why, when I had agreed... Why can't I get up? Why can't I get up? What is the reason? It's the third one. They're not going to meet these three; they have no discussion, just atomic thought. Each atomic idea is the master on the surface. You can't get the will; you can't actually have a conscience. You're not an individual.

This means the indiscriminate, which can not be separated. This means the division of the word "person" But we are separated, so we can't say we are individuals. We are only a divided crowd. Yoga is a person science. Yoga. This is how the individual is created, how this crowd becomes one, how a core can always be the master and how every slave can be put in his place. Then you need a detox of your mind; you need a catharsis- you need intense catharsis. You must throw out all that opposes you; you must turn your thoughts into peace. And don't allow a thing to come in because it's easy to allow, but then it's very difficult to move from there.

Therefore, the first thing in it is not to permit thoughts that do not help to create peace and then continue to seek and analyse what conflicting thoughts you have. Be the chosen. Stress the thoughts that can create inner harmony and inner quiet, then your mind will be purified. And you can see outside with this transparent body and you can go to a different body. The fourth, the fourth, is beyond the mental-body. The fourth body is known as the conscious mind body VIGYAN MAYKOS, because we don't know of any consciousness other than the mind, it will be impossible, difficult to distinguish between the subconscious physically and the conscious body. But if your subconscious is pure, you will simply realize that there is something else behind your mind, and your mind will be a door. Nevertheless, we can see....

You have feelings- it is one thing- but you can be sure of your emotions, and this consciousness is simply not a sensation. It's a sensation, a thought process. You've got frustration. You can be sure of this: "Actually, in me, there's a cycle of thinking, a mixture of emotions known as frustration, envy or love." You can stand out and understand that it's anger. You will say, "This is a thinking." This knowledge that this insight, this ability to observe the cycle of thinking, "this is a thought" produces the 4th body. Everyone therefore doesn't really have the fourth body created, but only as a possible. Only then will you have the fourth body when you become awake of your mind, and then there is creation. Sometimes we get observations, sometimes we get warning. When there is unexpected risk, disaster, a circumstance we haven't experienced before– we become conscious that the mind stops in that shock in the event of an accident for the first time. For example: If one drops a dagger suddenly in you, the mind ceases, because nothing can do or think. It's going to stop Thinking. And you become awake when thought ceases. You know the thinking has stopped, but there is still awareness: "I am alive".

It's the fourth heart, the body of our consciousness, our blood. We have it in a highly undeveloped way. It is difficult to develop, because there must be a lot of effort to stay mindful of each thought that goes through your mind. It is hard for you to remember any thought that has become an accumulation in your mind– one aspect of your mind, all the conditioning of the mind. It's hard, but not impossible. And you only have the right to be called a human being when this can happen; otherwise it is not. For an unconscious person means nothing. Then, impressions and ideas from abroad just throw you from here and there. You can't be swayed when you become awake! You are the alternative for the first time.

Buddha passed a village, and so many people came over to him with great exploit. They arrested him, beat him, and he threw stones at him. Then somebody asked, "What will you do now?" Buddha replied, "Nothing, I've become the chosen one now. You can't manipulate me; you can exploit me- that's your duty- but you can't react. It's not possible to manipulate me. It is just a trick if you misuse me and I react- and you can foresee the reaction. I'm not in it anymore. The button is pushed and there's light."

Reaction means you have not developed a conscious body, so you tend to react. However, such reactions, as you continue to respond, can not be defined as actions because actions only come with an aware that mature organism. You ACT then; if not, you must continue to respond. Someone is doing this, too you say it; somebody is doing it so and it's predictable. We assume he knows what will happen when the husband returns home in the evening. The whole scene can be foreseen: what would the wife ask?... He already knows the problem and intends answers now. And the wife already knows what he'll give answers. The entire game can be anticipated and repeated daily. What do we do? What do we do? The husband knows very well that whatever he says it won't be believed whatever he can say and yet he will respond in the same manner. The wife knows that whatever she asks, he will give the tricky reply, but still she continues to ask.

Are there talks? Unexpected. There's only a tricky game that they both play. And that's going on all their lives. People continue to react in the same old manner. How does this happen? When I know that if I ask that question, then I will give that answer; and when I'm aware, I don't need to ask. It's all absurd; it is not necessary to ask. And I asked for the same thing several times, and I was frustrated many times, and again. We're not even sure of it. As soon as the husband gets into the house, the issue arises, and the wife doesn't ask, it's mechanical. The question comes up, and the answer is used when there is a problem.

Have you always done anything as a conscious agent? No. No. If you did, you must have noticed something different from the mind. The consciousness of the mind, the consciousness of the cycle of thought, the fourth body standing outside the mind, outside, just as the spectator is an observer. The third is made up of thoughts; the fourth is made up of consciousness.

The fifth body is called the body of joy. This is the last, the body inside– but the body still. If the fourth corpus is purified, the fifth is realized if the fourth corpus is only transparent, as the fourth is then so transparent, that the fifth is directly felt. Therefore, you do not feel sleep, you feel happy, when you are in deep meditation. You feel not conscious, you feel happiness, when you are deep in meditation, when you are deeply aware. EOLBREAK If you start to feel joy, you are now conscious of that. The circumstance in which happiness is felt generates consciousness. Consciousness produces the fourth body's clarity and the fifth body. The fourth is made so clear that you can not only see it, you can pass it without any resistance– it is only a screen, it is simply an opening. The fourth body is the state of happiness. This happiness is there already. It can't be found anywhere, it can't be achieved, it can only be found. And by purifying the fourth body you discover it.

But this too is only a body and must be transcended; bliss must be transcended as well. You must go deeper, because you are still away from the center if you are unable to go beyond paradise. Since happiness is still an experience and it's still beyond the experiencer. So, whatever you hear, someone, this or that will belong to you. These five bodies are all experiences. And only the experiencer remains if there is no experience. Only the knowledge is left when there is no known entity.

You are focused around yourself if there is nothing to witness, but the only witness is, then you are; otherwise you are part of this or that entity. It's not an organ. This is the essence of the original. This is all being's spiritual source.

There are two or three more issues. You also transcend individuality as you transcend the joy- body. You also conquer life and death as you conquer the joy, for life and death are issues that only occur in the entity and the body. You can't die and not be resurrected if there's no body. So, once you know that the core does not exist for anyone, then there is no life or death– you are your own creation. Then you don't have personality, then you aren't. Every form and name have been lost. The process of purifying the fourth is meditation.

So, what should the fourth do? How to overcome it? How to overcoming it? How is joy transcended? It's hard to understand because we have absolutely no knowledge of happiness, so how to transcend is meaningless. One must first know, and you'll know the secret to transcend it when you do. The key is easily recognized because it's the last part. It's hard for everyone, because you face another body again. So, you go above one body, but you're stuck again within another body. When you get to the happy body, the next one is behind you and then there is no body behind the peace body for the first time. You are now close to the very center of life. Yet it has its own gravity: gravity is called grace. You throw something down and gravity, mm? The planet brings it away. The planet brings it away. But gravity can not operate beyond two hundred miles above ground. The moment the two hundred-mile barrier passes by a spacecraft, the earth can't pull it down. This is the tip of the pull of the world– 200 miles.

The body of happiness is only the beginning of the life of nobody. And you're on the move when you're in the blessed body. Now a new gravity begins to work, which is called gravity. That's why those who achieve the state beyond all bodies say, "We haven't reached it through our efforts; it's through God, and His grace." Actually, nothing can be done with the fifth. You just have to hit the fifth– that's the way to reach yourself. Go to the fifth and you are going to be pulled. It is always transcendence to achieve itself.

# Chapter Ten
# Conclusions

We lead common lives and don't know the latent divinity inside. We see them as our only reality, going through waking, dreaming and sleep states. Pujya Gurudevshri describes a fourth state of our consciousness while explaining the States and discusses how to manifest it for our spiritual enhancement.

The life of a human is described as the combination of three waking, dreaming and sleeping stages. You get up every morning and wake up, you get into the state of dreams when you go back at night and, when dreams stop, you get to the state of deep sleep. In this way, you spend your life, you have lived in those states since birth, and therefore you know these things.

In addition to these three nations, Turiya is the fourth member. This name does not have a specific name, unlike the first three called on the basis the state of body and mind. It's called Turiya as the fourth. Turiya is the fourth word. The condition can not be likened to the states of waking, dreaming and sleep which are considered to be states of the Self's ignorance. Turiya is a highly conscious state. In fact, this state is only achieved when one experiences the other three separately.

The consciousness waking state is whereby the soul, through senses and mind, knows the world of objects and thoughts. In the present condition, the mind and body function and interact with the outside world, but the knower, the Self, is not conscious. Apparently, the name of this state is an error. Just because you don't know any higher state, you see it as a waking state.

You know the world, but you don't really know who you are. You suggest that you've woken from sleep, but not if you don't know the Self. The day you wake up to the 4th state it is just another dream or a kind of sleep that you call the waking state.

The dream state of consciousness is where the soul encounters the world created by the mind without objects of contact etc. It is neither waking nor sleeping, nor understanding the Self. It's called a dream state because you're dreaming.

The mind is present here, but the body is not, because the senses are not aware of the outside world. The soul sees visions consisting of experiences of every day activity, hidden impulses or memories of past births. In this state, you see the reflections of objects, people and events of the waking world like a reflection from the moon in the water or object in a mirror. Holy people believe that man has a series of memories from endless past births in him. They're projected like a censor less movie. In visions you have no mental, actions or culture limitations, unlike waking states.

You never sense that you see a dream when dreaming. All feels "true." If you know that it's a dream as long as it's still on, then it's over and the waking has started.

There is no awareness of the outside world nor of the inner world of imagination in this third state of consciousness. Therefore, the word sleep is called the body, emotions and mind at rest. You don't feel things or reflections like dreams. It is said that this consciousness is deep in sleep. The non-self or the self is not understood.

To you, life is a series of non-self-alone experiences. You don't have the Self consciousness. You know the stone as well as pain but not yourself, for example, if a stone hurts your leg. You know the world of objects but not your real Self– the knower, the carrier of consciousness. You know what improvements are. You never remember the one who knows the case in the background of the situation. The soul goes across the three states and thus the states of the soul can be named, but in fact the soul is divided from the three states.

The Turiya (Fourth) State: The sages of yore are called the turiya state, a state of consciousness in which there is awareness of the learned. One can not reach the state of Turiya without being confident of one's true Self. When the experience in the self is intense, in each action, in all three states, an awareness of' I am,' the witness and the knower, remain constant.

You are associated with anything you see due to your unconsciousness of mind. In fact, you who see are free from everything you see. Like a dream, it all seems so real that you forget who you are and get involved. You remember it was only a dream when you woke up. But it tells you that there is a competent who flies across the three Nations. The fact that we recall dreaming Such nations aren't you, therefore. So soon as you become aware of the reality that you are separate from all these; the fourth condition starts to emerge. The Turiya Condition is mindful of supremacy.

How Can the Turiya State be Attained?

The experience of self-consciousness prevents the misrepresentation. Seek to differentiate from what comes and goes. It's hard because you identify with what you are not in endless lives and also have no practice of breaking this identity.

The illuminated people ask you to begin your waking practice. Start looking at yourself as the connoisseur. You may lose your identity with the non-self time and time again. Don't pause. Don't pause. Know yourself once more. Recall,' I'm not the doer, I'm only the knowing.' This consciousness will remain constant. You will be disturbed by memories from past lives. But if you keep reminding yourself as a knower with strong resolve and belief, every day it will be easier.

As you walk the path, focus moves from the seer. See the body walking; you're not driving. The focus moves from the task to the acquaintance during bathing. See that one bathes and knows the other. Know the flavour as a witness when feeding. See that one eats and only the other knows. Stay at home or at work, talk to someone and check– the know-how.

Do all things conscientiously– "All of this happens outside of myself. I am the experienced.' Keep up with that experience and increase awareness constantly. Even in your dream and sleep, you can slowly see this distinction.

As the consciousness rises, you will see that the thread of awareness also appears like a thread in pearls in and through the three states. You never will lose it because your fundamental nature is' to learn.' It was hidden from you until now, because you did not care about it and were accepted by what you saw. All you have to do is concentrate on the educated and the illusion will break down.

Wake Up!

He is truly successful who has just woven to the fourth stage. The others have just struggled with worldly possessions. He who has awaked throughout his life does not die again, because he has discovered that he is unborn, undying, invincible, everlasting and beyond the flesh.

Turiya State. Wake Up to it! Wake Up! Do so anywhere in the temple or on the street, wherever you can. The waking cycle is still the same. Be the informed and not the doer or the enjoyer of all things. Nobody can say how long it takes to achieve the state of Turiya. It depends all on your ability to be strong and your honesty. It can be just the moment. Because you don't have to go outside. It's just a matter of concentrating on yourself.

The depth of the sense of love, fulfilment and joy in the Turiya increases. You will sense harmony among all beings. The same lamp of consciousness in everyone you know. There is no friend, no foe, no mine, or yours to the awakened soul in the fourth state. Only an ocean of peace and happiness.

www.ingramcontent.com/pod-product-compliance
Lightning Source LLC
Chambersburg PA
CBHW072205100526
44589CB00015B/2382